A Nurse's Guide
to Caring for Elders

Mary Carroll, R.N., C, M.A., is a Certified Gerontological Nurse in private practice. She has held a wide variety of positions in acute, long-term, and home health care, and has presented numerous continuing education programs for health professionals. A member of Sigma Phi Omega, she serves on the board of the Central Illinois Chapter of the Alzheimer's Disease and Related Disorders Association.

L. Jane Brue, R.N., M.Ed., M.S.N., is an Assistant Professor of Nursing at Illinois Wesleyan University, Bloomington, Illinois. Her multifaceted nursing career includes having held the position of Director of Nursing in both acute and long-term care facilities. A member of Sigma Theta Tau, she has served on numerous district committees of the Illinois Nurses Association. She is also a board member of both the Corn Belt Chapter of the American Diabetic Association and the Bloomington–Normal Chapter of the Alzheimer's Disease and Related Disorders Association. Ms. Brue was selected to be a member of the Society of Nursing Professionals in *Who's Who in American Nursing*.

A Nurse's Guide to Caring for Elders

Mary Carroll, R.N., C, M.A.
L. Jane Brue, R.N., M.Ed., M.S.N.

SPRINGER PUBLISHING COMPANY
NEW YORK

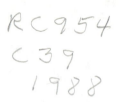

Springer Publishing Company, Inc.
536 Broadway
New York, NY 10012

88 89 90 91 92 / 5 4 3 2 1

Library of Congress Cataloging-in-Publication Data

Carroll, Mary, R.N.
  A nurse's guide to caring for elders.

  Includes bibliographies and index.
  1. Geriatric nursing. I. Brue, L. Jane.
II. Title. [DNLM: 1. Geriatric Nursing. 2. Nursing
Process. WY 152 C319n]
RC954.C39 1987   610.73'65   87-26593
ISBN 0-8261-5520-0 (soft)

Printed in the United States of America

Contents

v

MAY 5 1988

PART III   Focusing on the Whole Person

Acknowledgments

The authors wish to express their appreciation to those who have given their support to this project. Our husbands, Jim Carroll and John Brue, deserve special mention for their understanding of the work involved. Special recognition must be given to Gari Lesnoff-Caravaglia, Ph.D., of the Center on Aging, University of Massachusetts. Without her wisdom this text could not have been written.

The authors also wish to thank their colleagues and the many older persons who contributed to our combined clinical experience of over 50 years. Jerry D. Durham, Ph.D., of Illinois Wesleyan University, Bloomington, Illinois, is especially acknowledged for his contribution on the psychosocial aspects of older persons. We are also grateful to Dalisey Bello-Manabat, M.D., and Gregorio Manabat, M.D., for their expert assistance with aspects of this book that involve medical practice, and sincerely appreciate the help of Ralph Bellas, Ph.D., and Louise Bellas, M.S.N., with the copyediting.

Introduction

The care of older persons is possibly the most complex area in nursing. It is also an area characterized by the most rapid growth. Sociologists predict that by the year 2000 persons 65 and older will represent 13% to 15% of the population. Five percent of the older population (65 years and older) live in long-term care facilities, with the remaining 95% residing in the community. As a result of the increased life-span of older persons, there is a sharp increase in the number of elders requiring health care. Thus, a renewed emphasis on gerontological nursing is evolving. According to recent figures, hospitals account for 67% of registered nurse employment in the United States, while nursing homes employ 7.7%, community/public health employs 6.8%, and ambulatory care employs 6.6% ("R.N. employment," 1986). However, these data probably underestimate the percentages of nurses employed in long-term care, community/public health, and ambulatory facilities, since this data was gathered prior to full implementation of the Prospective Payment System (PPS). Implementation of the PPS has resulted in earlier discharge from acute care facilities, creating a burgeoning home health industry. The trend toward increased care in the home is reflected in this volume, which has been designed to serve nurses in both institutional and home settings. Nurses in extended care and home health agencies are challenged to care for persons who are more acutely ill and require complex nursing services. These nurses need special clinical skills as well as communication skills, the ability to use the nursing process effectively, and, most importantly, a love and respect for older persons, which is essential to the provision of quality nursing care.

Gerontological nursing is complicated by the fact that older persons usually have multiple health problems and that there are more individual differences among older persons than any other age group. All persons age at different rates—many persons of advanced age are functioning well and are in good health, while some younger persons are totally dependent on others for their care. It is necessary to have an understanding of the differences in function that occur with aging in order to facilitate the application of the nursing process.

In the past, the focus of traditional medicine has been on the treatment of disease. Now, however, there is a national trend toward wellness-oriented health care, disease prevention, and health promotion. Gerontological nurses are in an excellent position to assist older persons to achieve wellness through functional assessment and supportive-educative nursing interventions.

This book is intended to provide the nurse with essential information for treating the common health problems found in the elderly in a brief, easy-to-use format. Nursing diagnoses are integrated throughout. In addition to discussing all basic categories of health problems, the book addresses general principles of promoting wellness, including psychosocial considerations, nutrition, and the creation of a facilitative environment to enhance an elder's quality of life.

Briefly, Chapter 1 begins with the first step in the nursing process—the initial interview and health history. A detailed "Subjective Assessment Worksheet" is provided as a sample interview tool. Chapter 2 provides information about normal age-related changes commonly seen in older persons and describes how to perform a physical assessment. The physical assessment is approached from the perspective of a "head to toe" review of systems. An in-depth physical assessment guide is also provided.

In Chapters 3 through 11 various potential health problems and common pathological conditions of elders are discussed. Each chapter contains a description of potential health problems, followed by examples of potential nursing diagnoses and potential nursing interventions related to the diagnostic statement. Occasionally nursing considerations are cited when information of particular importance is relevant to the potential health problem.

Chapters 12, 13, and 14 provide information that focuses on the whole person—psychosocial, nutritional, and environmental aspects. Chapter 15 offers guidance on developing a plan of care. Chapter 16 allows the reader to synthesize and evaluate the information in five case studies. The case studies provide examples of older people in acute care, extended care, and home health care settings. This chapter includes "Learning Vignettes"—sample cases from which readers can develop their own nursing diagnoses and interventions.

"Learning Checks" are included at the conclusion of each chapter for use in evaluation of learning. The Appendixes contain the American Nurses' Association's (ANA) Standards of Gerontological Nursing and the answers to the "Learning Checks" and the "Learning Vignettes."

It is the author's intent that *A Nurse's Guide to Caring for Elders* will be useful for all nurses, students, or practitioners who care for older persons.

REFERENCE

R.N. employment: The latest trends. (1986). *Chart, 86*(6), 3.

Contributor

Jerry D. Durham, R.N., Ph.D., the contributor of the chapter on "Psychosocial Aspects of Elders' Care," is Director of the School of Nursing, Illinois Wesleyan University, Bloomington, Illinois. A prolific author, Dr. Durham also maintains a private practice in mental health nursing.

PART I
First Steps of the Nursing Process

The purposes of Part I are to:
1. *Define aging in physiological terms*
2. *Present an overview of the physiologic changes that occur as part of the normal aging process*
3. *Provide a guide for collecting the health history and accomplishing the physical assessment of older persons*

1

The Initial Interview and Health History

The collection of the health history is the first step in the subjective nursing assessment. The purposes of this procedure are to establish rapport and communication, to determine the person's expectations of nursing, and to gather data for the formulation of nursing diagnoses and of a plan of care. The history is best collected *prior* to admission to the long-term care facility or health care agency in order to provide adequate planning for the potential client's needs. A multidisciplinary team (i.e., nursing and social services personnel) may visit the person; however, the team should not include more than two or three members to avoid overwhelming the older person. Since nursing is the keystone of long-term care, a registered nurse must participate in the initial interview and assessment. Each discipline has its own information needs, although these frequently overlap. The various health care disciplines should determine what information will be obtained by whom to avoid redundancy in the interview. Representatives from each discipline should interview the client privately, whenever possible. Following the initial interview by the various team members, a multidisciplinary conference is held to plan for the client's care.

The visit may take place in the client's home, in an acute care hospital, in another health care agency, or in the long-

term care facility. The time for the interview should be predetermined, and the spouse, children, and/or significant others
should be present, if possible. If the person is acutely ill or
has a verbal or auditory communication deficit, it is imperative that another person be present to assist the prospective
client. The focus of the interview always remains on the client.

Care must be taken not to overtax a person who is weak or
acutely ill. Often a great deal of the necessary information
can be obtained with the client's permission from the hospital medical record, or from the plans of care of other nursing
agencies who have cared for the individual. Any information
from other sources needs to be confirmed. Medical jargon
should be avoided in the interview; the person should express the health problem in his or her own terms. Additionally, the client should be addressed as Mr. _____ , Mrs.
_____ , or Miss _____ , unless he or she indicates
a personal preference to be called by the first name. Names
such as "Honey," "Sweetie," "Gramps," and "Granny"
should never be used. Only pertinent information need be
collected during the initial interview. For example, there is no
point in eliciting a detailed history of childhood illnesses if
there is no relationship to the current problem or reason for
admission, since such information can usually be obtained
from other sources. The nursing history should focus on the
principal health problem(s) of the individual, that is, the rea-
son(s) for seeking nursing care. In addition to a detailed assessment of the reason(s), the initial health history should
also include self-care practices, the medication history, and
basic nutrition history. The interview should also focus on
the person's strengths, what abilities are intact, and the person's expectations; for example, the person's desire (or lack
of desire) to relearn ambulation following a stroke. However,
the reason for seeking care is always due to a health problem,
and it is often difficult to identify strengths when the per-

son's physical problems are severe. Self-care practices are often examples of the older person's assets.

The nurse can also accomplish a general inspection during the initial interview. Areas that can be easily evaluated are the person's ability to ambulate, with or without assistance or assistive devices; and the ability to accomplish activities of daily living (ADLs), such as eating, drinking, transferring, toileting, and dressing. Obvious pain or lack of pain and the state of mental awareness should also be recorded. The nurse can also assess skin color, the existing state of personal hygiene, and the person's relationship to his or her surroundings and significant others.

The medication history should note the drugs currently prescribed including dosage, route, time of administration, and if the person takes a food or beverage with the medication, as well as any drug allergies and untoward reactions the person might have experienced. The history should also include drugs that have been discontinued, since high blood levels of such drugs can persist due to age-related alterations in absorption, distribution, and excretion times. Discontinued medication can provide clues to health problems the person may not identify, such as hypertension, infections, and epilepsy, among others.

A history of over-the-counter (OTC) medication, including skin ointments and topically applied medication, needs to be taken. The person should be asked what remedies he or she takes, or what measures are taken for the relief of muscle/joint pain, headache, gastrointestinal discomfort, including constipation and diarrhea, and insomnia. If the person is to enter a long-term care facility, the nurse must be aware of the facility's policies and procedures for obtaining and dispensing drugs, and consult the pharmacist if there is any question about procuring the necessary medication.

Basic information about nutrition should include the person's ability to feed himself or herself, chew, and swallow.

The nurse should note if the person receives a prescribed therapeutic diet, or if he or she maintains a particular self-determined diet, and the person's usual meal times. The nurse inquires about any food allergies, intolerances, or dietary practices prescribed by the person's religious persuasion or ethnic group. Any vitamins, food supplements, or health foods normally used should also be noted.

The interview should be terminated whenever the person appears to tire, lose interest, or is in pain. The remainder of the health history, including the family, past illnesses, and immunization histories (including influenza and pneumonia vaccinations) can be collected during subsequent interviews. This information is often required by licensing agencies.

Even though the person may be advanced in years, the past family history (parents, siblings, grandparents) can be of value in anticipating potential health problems. Similarly, the health history of the person's offspring can be used to identify potential health problems, such as familial tendencies toward cardiovascular problems or diabetes.

The health history is completed by noting past illnesses, surgery, hospitalizations, and any other health problems. Responses should be recorded at the time they are given; the nurse should verbally paraphrase or repeat any responses that seem unclear.

Unfortunately, it is not always possible to complete the history and initial nursing assessment prior to admission or utilization of services, although every effort to accomplish this must be made. In the hospital and nursing home setting, the initial assessment is made at the time of admission. The nurse must spend the greatest amount of time orienting the person to the new environment, establishing communication and rapport, and relieving anxiety. When only the principal health problem is dealt with, the patient should be informed as to when the nurse will return to complete the data collection and assessment. In the home health setting, it is most ideal if the initial interview can be accomplished before discharge from the acute care facility.

Any health information forwarded from other agencies and health care personnel should be carefully reviewed. Nurses should not hesitate to consult with other nurses who have cared for the person. Unfortunately, consultation with other members of the nursing profession is sometimes overlooked as a valuable resource for planning and providing care.

It is important that the nurse who conducts the initial interview continue the data collection to maintain rapport, communication, and trust, as well as to review, validate, and perhaps revise information from the initial interview. If this is impossible, the original nurse should introduce the nurse who will complete the data collection, and the information from the first interview should be reviewed with the person and the new nurse.

A suggested subjective assessment worksheet for the collection of the health history is provided (pp. 8–28).

SUBJECTIVE ASSESSMENT WORKSHEET

SECTION 1
BIOGRAPHICAL DATA BASE

1. CLIENT PROFILE

single _____
Name: _____ Sex: _____ Race: _____married _____
divorced _____
widowed _____
separated _____

Address: _____

Telephone: _____

Birthplace: _____ Birthdate: _____

Age (at last birthday): _____

Religion: _____ Ethnic background: _____

Occupation (if retired, before retirement): _____

Satisfaction with present or past employment:

Education: _____ Nearest contact person: _____

2. FAMILY PROFILE

Spouse:
_____ living
    health status:
    age:
    occupation:

_____ deceased
    year deceased:
    cause of death:

Children:

_____ living (name, sex, age, and place of residence):

_____ deceased (name, sex, year deceased, cause of death):

Others in household:

Relationship with family or significant others:

3. HOME PROFILE

Type: _____

Ownership or rent status: _____

Size in relation to need: _____

Accessibility to and mobility within: _____

_____

_____

Safety features: _____

_____

_____

Management of maintenance and repair: _____

_____

Adequacy of heating, lighting, ventilation, water: _____

_____

_____

Important objects in environment: _____

_____

Pets and plants: _____

Nearest neighbor: _____

4. COMMUNITY PROFILE

Knowledge of community resources (transportation, recreation/social, shopping, health care, church, other):

_____

_____

Availability of community resources: _____

_____

_____

Use of community resources: _____

_____

Accessibility to community resources: _____

_____

Safety provisions: _____

5. ECONOMIC PROFILE

Sources: Retirement income: _____

          Social Security: _____

          Other: _____

Perception of adequacy (present or anticipated): _____

_____

Management of cost of health care (medication, supplies, transportation, services):

_____ Medicare   _____ Food stamps

_____ Medicaid   _____ Supplementary insurance

6. HEALTH RESOURCES CURRENTLY USED

_____ Private M.D.   _____ H.M.O.   _____ Mobile meals

_____ Hospital   _____ Public health nurse

_____ Clinic   _____ Social worker

Other:

SECTION 2
HEALTH PERCEPTION–HEALTH MANAGEMENT PATTERN
COGNITIVE–PERCEPTION PATTERN
COPING–STRESS TOLERANCE PATTERN

1. Personal perception of current health status (feeling of well-being):

_____ Excellent   _____ Fair

_____ Good   _____ Poor

(May rate self on a scale of 1 to 10 with 10 being excellent.)

2. Current health status:
   Knowledge and understanding of health problem:

   Limitation(s) of function or performance of Activities of Daily Living (ADL):

Management of limitation(s):

Health goals:

3. Immunizations (include date received):

Tetanus: _____   Pneumonia: _____
Influenza: _____   Other: _____

4. Allergies (describe agent and reaction to foods, drugs, contact substances, environmental factors):

5. Health examinations:

EXAM	DATE	M.D./CLINIC	FINDINGS	INSTRUCTIONS
Physical				
Dental				
Vision				
Hearing				
Breast				
Pap smear or prostate				
Occult blood (Guaiac test)				
Chest x-ray				
TB test				
Pulmonary function				

6. Past health status (serious or chronic illnesses)

	Yes	*No*	*Date*		*Yes*	*No*	*Date*
Arthritis				Hepatitis			
Cataracts				Pneumonia			
Diabetes				Seizure disorder			
Glaucoma				Thyroid disease			
Heart Disease				Tuberculosis			
Hypertension				Kidney disease			
Ulcer				Other			
Liver disease							

7. Hospitalizations/operations:

Procedure/Condition	*Date*	*Reason*	*Duration of stay*
_____	_____	_____	_____
_____	_____	_____	_____
_____	_____	_____	_____
_____	_____	_____	_____

8. Current medications (prescription and OTC)

Name	Dosage	Frequency	Date ordered	Knowledge & understanding	Exp. date

9. Family history (use diagrammatic   Key: Male
   format and include current illnesses):   Female
                                                    Deceased (state
                                                    cause of death)

10. Activities to ensure personal safety:

    _____ Never walk alone at night

    _____ Lock car, home

    _____ Carry objects for self-defense (describe)

    _____ Acquire self-defense skills (describe)

    _____ Wear seatbelt while driving/riding in car

    _____ Carry identification on person in case of emergency:

        Blood type_____   Allergy to penicillin_____

        Diabetic_____   Seizures_____

11. Habits with potential to alter health:

    Smoking: Type (pipes, cigar, cigarette, other):

                       Quantity:

                       Duration:

                       Inhale?

                       Increase when anxious/stressed?

                       Desire to quit?

    Drinking: Type of alcohol:

                       Frequency/amount per day/week:

                       Increase when anxious/stressed?

    Caffeine: Coffee   Tea   Soft drinks

                       Frequency/amount per day:

                       Increase when anxious/stressed?

    Personal habits:

_____ Regularly listen to loud music or watch TV

_____ Read with inadequate light source

_____ Use aerosol sprays

_____ Sunbathe without skin protection or hat

_____ Others (describe)

12. Environmental precautionary measures:

_____ Avoid overloading electrical circuits

_____ Keep emergency numbers posted near phone (fire dept., police, hospital, family)

_____ Proper storage of medicines and chemical agents

_____ Avoid keeping combustible materials stored in home/apt.

_____ Avoid throw rugs

_____ Have sufficient, non-glaring light

_____ Avoid temperature extremes

_____ Smoke detector in home/apt.

_____ Safety bars in bathroom tub/shower

13. Sensory status (describe degree of limitation and assistive measures):

Hearing:

  All sounds:

  High frequencies:

Vision:

  Full vision: Color discrimination:

  Night vision: Depth perception:

  Peripheral vision: Reading:

Taste: Adequacy:

Smell: Adequacy:

Touch:

    Feel pressure & pain:

    Different temperatures:

Speech:

14. Assistive devices:

    Hearing aid: Contact lenses: Glasses:

    Telephone amplifier:

    Other:

15. Cognitive status:

    Memory (recent and remote):

    Perceived difficulty learning:

    Easiest way to learn things:

16. Emotional status: Client self-perception*

    _____ Anxious   _____ Bored   _____ Fearful

    _____ Depressed   _____ Tense   _____ Suspicious

    When (if) you have a big problem (any problem) in your life, how do you handle it?

    Do you handle everyday problems as well as most persons your age?

17. Client's description of a typical day:

_____

*Please note if different from interviewer's perception

SECTION 3
NUTRITION–METABOLIC PATTERN
SKIN INTEGRITY

1. What is your usual daily food intake (use 24-hour diet recall and include fluids):

	FOOD EATEN	AMOUNT	CALORIES	TIME OF DAY

BREAKFAST

_____

_____

_____

_____

_____

LUNCH

_____

_____

_____

_____

_____

SUPPER

_____

_____

_____

_____

FOOD EATEN   AMOUNT   CALORIES   TIME OF DAY

SNACKS

_____

_____

_____

Total calories _____

2. Special preferences or prescribed restrictions in relation to food/fluid intake:

3. Description of appetite:

4. Companionship during mealtime:

5. Ability to buy and prepare food:

6. Ability to read labels on foods purchased:

7. Ability to swallow and chew different types of food:

8. Use of food supplements (vitamins, minerals, liquids):

9. Client satisfied with present weight?

10. Knowledge of "Basic 4," caloric requirements for age:

11. Client's self-evaluation of nutritional status:

12. Circle: indigestion, nausea, vomiting, abdominal pain, gas. Describe factors that precipitate symptom and measures that relieve the symptom.

13. Which of the following dietary practices apply to client? (circle letter)

    a. Uses daily vitamin/mineral supplement
    b. Uses antacids frequently
    c. Eats in slow, relaxed manner

    d. Eats candy or other sweets
    e. Eats even when not hungry
    f. Adds salt to food
    g. Reads labels on food
    h. Avoids foods with sugar added
    i. Avoids refined or processed foods
    j. Maintains ideal weight within 10 lbs.
    k. Skips meals
    l. Nibbles food all day
    m. Uses salt/sugar substitutes

SKIN, NAILS, HAIR

1. Skin care practices:

   Protection from sun:

   Use of creams or oils:

   Frequency of bathing:

   Soaps used:

2. Occurrence of skin lesions, bruises, or bleeding:

3. Care of skin lesions:

4. Changes in characteristics or color of skin (especially extremities):

5. Skin condition:

   _____ Dry   _____ Moist   _____ Pigmentation changes

6. Nail care practices:

   frequency of cutting:
   method of cutting:
   ability to cut nails:

7. Hair care practices:
   Ability to care for hair: _____
   Changes in texture, thickness, color: _____
   Methods used for hair care—use of dyes: _____
   Wears wig: _____

SECTION 4
ELIMINATION PATTERNS

BLADDER

1. How often do you urinate in a 24-hour period?

2. Have you taken a medication that has affected your urine? If yes, describe.

3. What activities do you perform to maintain your urinary elimination? Do you always respond to the urge to urinate? Are you able to stop the flow of urine at will?

4. Do you or have you ever practiced exercises to strengthen bladder or pelvic muscles?

5. How do you care for the environment to maintain sanitary conditions?

6. Describe your urine in terms of color, quantity, odor, clarity:

7. Associated factors:

   _____ Change in stream of urination   _____ Pus in urine

   _____ Stress incontinence   _____ Nocturia

   _____ Excessive secretion of urine   _____ Urinary frequency

   _____ Decrease in urinary output   _____ Urinary infection

   _____ Dribbling or incontinence

BOWEL

1. What is the usual time and frequency of defecation?

2. Describe stools in terms of color, odor, shape, and consistency.

3. Use of digestive or evacuation aids (include name, frequency of use, and results):

4. What activities are performed to maintain bowel elimination?

5. Do you always respond to the urge to have a bowel movement? When do you not respond?

6. How do you care for the environment to maintain sanitary conditions?

7. Associated factors (describe practices used to aid if these conditions occur):

_____ Diarrhea

_____ Constipation

_____ Hemorrhoids

_____ Bleeding

_____ Straining

SECTION 5
ACTIVITY–EXERCISE PATTERN
SLEEP–REST PATTERN

1. Describe social/leisure activities (include membership in organizations, hobbies, and interests):

2. Is there sufficient energy for desired/required activities?

3. What is the degree of independence for the activity? Of satisfaction with independence?

4. Self-rating of physical fitness: On what basis?

   Excellent _____ Good _____ Fair _____ Poor _____

5. Describe exercise program(s) (type, frequency):

   Do you check pulse rate before, during, or after exercise?

6. Mobility status:

   _____ Ambulatory _____ Nonambulatory

   _____ Ambulatory with assistance (specify aids used)

   　　Degree of confidence in using mobility aids:

   　　Reactions to use of aids:

   　　Knowledge of proper use and maintenance of aids:

   _____ Able to climb stairs

   _____ Able to rise from chair, toilet

7. Extremity function (circle those that apply)—describe location, degree of limitation, and assistive measures:

   Contracture:

   Painful movement:

   Paralysis:

   Spasm:

   Amputation:

8. Perceived ability for: (Code for level*)

   _____ Feeding _____ Grooming

   _____ Bathing _____ General mobility

_____ Toileting   _____ Cooking

_____ Bed mobility _____ Home maintenance

_____ Dressing   _____ Shopping

*Functional level codes
Level 0:   Full self-care
Level I: Requires use of equipment or device
Level II: Requires assistance or supervision from another
Level III: Requires assistance or supervision from another and equipment
            or device
Level IV: Is dependent and does not participate

9. Circulation (circle those that apply)—describe   precipitating factors, degree of limitation, and relief measures:

   Chest pain:

   Tachycardia:

   Edema:

   Cramping in extremities:

SLEEP

10. Type of bed:

    Sleep alone or with another:

11. Describe usual sleep pattern (retiring hour, arising hour, number of hours
    of sleep—include naps):

12. Practices that promote going to sleep (include drugs or routines):

13. If you do not feel rested upon awakening, what do you do to correct this
    occurrence?

BREATHING

14. Describe your breathing pattern:

15. What promotes or impedes your lung expansion?

16. Describe any breathing exercises you perform and your purpose for doing them.

17. What causes a change in your usual breathing pattern?

18. What practices do you engage in when your breathing pattern is altered? (Include use of medications for allergy or breathing problems)

19. What do you do to maintain a clean air environment for yourself?

20. Screen for (circle those that apply)

_____ Orthopnea   _____ Dyspnea

_____ Shortness of breath _____Wheezing

_____ Cough

21. Sputum characteristics (describe):

SECTION 6
ROLE–RELATIONSHIP PATTERN
COPING–STRESS TOLERANCE PATTERN
SELF-PERCEPTION—SELF-CONCEPT PATTERN
SEXUALITY–REPRODUCTIVE PATTERN
VALUE–BELIEF PATTERN

It may be useful to review the biographical data assessment prior to beginning this assessment.

1. Do you have difficulty handling family problems?

2. Do you visit with relatives and friends as often as you want?

3. Do things generally go well for you in your relationships?

4. Do you feel adequate in group situations? What would you like to change, anything?

5. Describe the kind and amount of alone time you have (note perceived adequacy):

6. Do you have feelings of loneliness and how are they managed?

7. Describe any recent changes in your life style (i.e., divorce, moving, new job, family illness, financial stress):

8. Is there someone whom you can trust and confide in?

9. Do you feel part of (or isolated in) your living unit, neighborhood, city, etc?

10. History of counseling? Describe nature of counseling.

MENTAL STATUS

1. How would you describe yourself in a few sentences?

2. Describe how you think others perceive you. (Consistent/inconsistent with self-description?)

3. What things make you feel good about yourself, bad about yourself?

4. Affect (usual mood, factors that affect mood):

5. Perceptions of self in relation to age:

6. Perceptions of self-appearance (include any changes noted, importance of appearance):

7. Do you find things frequently make you angry? annoyed? fearful? depressed? Describe fully. What helps?

8. What do you do if another does not approve of your actions, beliefs, values?

SEXUALITY–REPRODUCTIVE PATTERNS

9. Are your needs for affection being met?

10. Self-description of relationships with members of the same sex:

11. Self-description of relationships with members of the opposite sex:

12. Birth control measures practiced? Did you take birth control pills?

13. *Female* reproductive factors:

    _____ Vaginal discharge

    _____ Itching

    _____ Lesions

    _____ Breast mass

    _____ Nipple discharge

    _____ Breast pain

    _____ Mastectomy (R or L)

    _____ Prosthesis

    _____ Breast self-examination (note frequency, method). If no, explain why not.

14. Postmenopausal or climacteric difficulties:

15. Use of hormones or other medications related to sexual organs:

16. *Male* reproductive factors:

    _____ Scrotal swelling

    _____ Lesions

_____ Discharge

_____ Prostate problems

_____ Penis and scrotum self-examination practices (note frequency, method). If no, explain why not.

_____ Use of condoms for prevention of infectious diseases

VALUE–BELIEF PATTERNS

17. Do you generally get the things you want out of life?

18. What are your plans for future?

19. Describe attitudes and concerns about death:

20. Self-description of importance of religion in life:

21. Religious affiliations:

    Opportunity to attend religious services:

    Ability to attend religious services:

    Contact with clergy:

    Importance of religious programs on TV or radio:

    Significance of religious holidays, observance of:

LEARNING CHECK

1. The health history and initial interview are best recorded _____ to admission.

2. The initial interview should focus on the person's _____ _____ _____ .

3. In addition to the evaluation of the principal health problem, _____ and _____ histories need to be determined during the initial interview.

4. The purposes of the initial interview are to gather health data, establish rapport, and facilitate communication to determine _____ _____ _____ .

5. The interview should be _____ whenever the person appears to tire, lose interest, or is in pain.

6. In the home health setting, it is most ideal if the initial interview is accomplished _____ _____ from the acute care facility.

7. In the hospital or nursing home setting, the nurse _____ spends time orienting the person to a new environment, establishing _____ , and _____ _____ .

8. During the interview, the nurse should _____ or _____ any responses that seem unclear.

2

The Physical Changes of Aging and How to Assess Them

Various licensure regulations require that a physical examination be completed and recorded by a physician within a given time period associated with the admission to acute and long-term care facilities. The nurse needs to review the findings of the examination and note any parts that may have been deferred. Therefore, it may not be necessary for the nurse to perform a complete physical examination initially. In the home health setting, it is also necessary to have a statement of health.

The physical assessment performed by the nurse may be very lengthy and thorough or may focus only on the principal problem and general condition of the person. The purposes of the assessment are to further enhance communication and rapport and to obtain baseline information about the health status of the older person. The assessment must not be hurried; the procedure must be explained, privacy must be maintained, and the environment kept sufficiently warm to protect the person from chilling.

The following material discusses normal age changes commonly manifested in older persons. These normal age changes are addressed in the basic strategies of the physical assessment, which are inspection, palpation, percussion, and auscultation. *Inspection* involves the systematic observation of the body through the special senses of sight, hearing, smell, and touch. Eliopoulos (1984) pointed out that a great deal can be assessed through odors emitted from the client. Excessive use of perfumes can be associated with poor sense of smell, breath odor may indicate lung abscesses and infections in the mouth, and an odor of newly mown clover may indicate liver failure (p. 301). *Palpation* involves touching the body surfaces with the hands or fingers to identify temperature, texture, organ location, and size. *Percussion* is the tapping of specific body areas to determine information about underlying tissue. *Auscultation* involves listening to body sounds with a stethoscope. The evaluation of the various organ systems may be done in any order.

HEAD AND NECK

It is usually most convenient to begin the physical assessment with the evaluation of the head and neck. The head is inspected for gross lesions and asymmetry. Visual acuity decreases with advancing age. Peripheral vision and color vision decrease. The warm colors such as orange and yellow can be seen better than blues and greens. There is increased sensitivity to glare, and increased adjustment time to changes in light intensities. The eyes are observed for swelling, redness, excessive tearing, or dryness. The eyelids are observed for lesions and encrustations. The iris of the eye is inspected for the presence/absence of an arcus senilis, a whitish ring around the cornea. The size of the pupils is noted. The pupillary reaction to light can be evaluated with a pen light. Vision may be checked with the Snellen chart or test, or by asking the person to read printed material or to describe a picture or article on a wall. Cataracts can be identified by shining the pen light at a 45° angle to the eye. Cloudy opacities are seen if cataracts are present.

A fundoscopic exam may be performed if the examiner has the necessary skills and equipment. The nurse is referred to the text by Bates (1983) for a complete description of the fundoscopic exam.

Major changes in hearing include less perception of high frequency tones. It becomes more difficult to discriminate sounds when there is more than one sound being received. Carotenuto and Bullock (1981) state that there is a decrease in cerumen production with age.

The external ears are inspected for symmetry, lesions, and any obvious drainage. The lower lobe should be observed for a longitudinal fold, which may indicate cardiovascular disease. The internal ear may be visualized with an otoscope. A cone of light should be visualized on the eardrum. The ear canal should be inspected for accumulations of impacted cerumen and scarring from previous infections, which may cause hearing loss.

Hearing is tested by standing behind the person, pronouncing two-syllable words, and asking the person to repeat the words as they are enunciated. If the person uses a hearing aid, the hearing should be assessed with and without the hearing aid.

The Weber and Rinne tests may also be performed. The Weber test is done by striking a tuning fork and then pressing the stem of the fork against the skull in the center of the head. The sound should be heard equally in both ears. The person should be asked if the sound is louder in either ear.

The Rinne test is done by striking a tuning fork and then placing the stem of the fork on the mastoid bone. When the person can no longer hear the sound, the fork is placed near the auditory meatus. The sound should again be heard. Normally air conduction (AC) is greater than bone conduction (BC). This is expressed as $AC > BC$. The older adult will frequently have some hearing loss, most commonly due to presbycusis, which is a loss due to changes in the inner ear structure.

The nose and nostrils are observed for obvious deviation and drainage. The ability to smell is tested by asking the person to identify the smell of an alcohol swab or another pungent odor while the eyes are closed. A decline in the ability to smell occurs with aging.

In the oral cavity of an older person, the teeth become worn as a result of abrasions of the enamel and dentin. There is decreased production of saliva and shrinkage of the gums. According to Bennett, Creamer, and Fontana-Smith (1981, p. 108), the major cause of loss of teeth in older persons is periodontal disease. The oral cavity is carefully inspected for dentition and condition of the mucosa. Any foul odors are noted, since breath odor can indicate various health problems. If the person has dentures, they are observed for proper fit, cleanliness, and occlusion. The gums and periodontal tissue are examined for color, moisture, presence/absence of lesions, and infections. Any broken teeth or teeth in poor repair are noted, as well as the state of dental hygiene.

The entire head and neck are gently palpated for tenderness, sores, enlarged nodes. The thyroid gland, which is located across the trachea below the cricoid cartilage, is palpated. The gland is often easier to palpate if the person is asked to swallow.

SKIN/INTEGUMENT

Loss of subcutaneous fat and elasticity resulting in wrinkling of the skin occurs with advancing age. Sweat glands decrease in activity and number. Sometimes pigment cells hypertrophy, causing hyperpigmentation or "liver spots." Blood supply to the skin and the capillaries become more fragile due to the loss of supporting subcutaneous fat. Hair thins and hair roots atrophy. The nails become thicker and more brittle, and their growth is slowed.

The skin is observed for color, presence or absence of lesions, moisture, and/or dryness. The frequency of cherry angiomas increases with aging, but the significance of this type of lesion is unknown. The nails are observed for evidence of clubbing, discoloration, and splitting. The skin and nails are also observed for general cleanliness and odor. The breasts are inspected for symmetry, dimpling, and inversion of the nipples, which signifies breast pathology.

The skin is also assessed by gentle touch for temperature, texture, and turgor. Turgor is best assessed by gently raising or moving the skin of the forehead and observing how rapidly the crease disappears or returns to normal. Any lesions should be described in terms of size, which is determined by measurement; color; presence or absence of hair; induration; and pain or numbness.

Special attention should be given to the feet. They must be carefully inspected for any lesions, especially in the areas between the toes. The examiner must also note any corns, calluses, ulcers, warts, bunions, or hammer toe deviations. The toenails are observed for cleanliness, color, abnormal thickening, or fungal infections. Nails grow more slowly in the older adult.

RESPIRATORY SYSTEM

The respiratory system undergoes the greatest age-associated change and decrease in function, even though lung tissue regenerates well. Stretch and muscle tone of the chest wall decrease, as do all the muscles associated with respiration. The ribs become less mobile, and the costal cartilage calcifies. There is decreased action of the cilia, dilation of the bronchioles, and a decrease in the number of alveoli. The cough reflex and cough effectiveness are reduced. These changes result in reduced depth of respiration, decreased ventilation, and decreased vital capacity, which Armstrong and Cleary

(1982, p. 2) state is the most accurate predictor of the general health of older persons. These changes result in reduced oxygenation of all body tissues. When interpreting arterial blood gas (ABG) values, 1 mm Hg for every year of age over 60 to age 90 should be subtracted from the PaO value ("Interpreting Arterial Blood Gases," 1980).

Inspection of the respiratory system should be done with the person seated in a chair to observe for symmetrical chest expansion. The shape of the chest, any skeletal deformities, and respiratory effort are observed.

The index and third fingers are run along the spinal column to determine any abnormal curvature. Diaphragmatic excursion is evaluated by grasping the rib cage with both hands, with the thumbs at the level of the 10th ribs near the spine. The movement of the thumbs is observed while the person inhales deeply. Movement of the thumbs should be equal and symmetrical. Tactile fremitus is evaluated by placing the side or palm of the dominant hand at the right scapular area, and asking the person to say "99." The hand is then moved to the left scapular area and progressively down the back alternating sides. The person repeats "99" each time the hand is moved. The vibrations palpated should feel equal.

Percussion should always be done very gently. The entire posterior chest is percussed, except the scapular areas where bony structures overlie lung tissue. Resonance should be equal on both sides of the chest. The flat large diaphragm of the stethoscope is used to listen to the lungs while the person breathes deeply with the mouth open. The auscultation must be done slowly to avoid hyperventilation. The lungs should sound clear with no adventitious or abnormal sounds. Rales sound like a lock of hair rubbed between the fingers near the ear. Rhonchi are continuous deeper sounds caused by obstructions to the air flow. Wheezes are high-pitched whistling sounds caused by partial airway obstruction.

CARDIOVASCULAR SYSTEM

The respiratory system and cardiovascular system are closely related. A change in one system directly affects the other. The heart muscle becomes stiffer and less compliant with age. Increased rigidity and thickening occur in the heart valves, and efficiency of blood return to the heart decreases. The aorta becomes less elastic and enlarges and elongates. Coronary circulation decreases. Carotenuto and Bullock (1980) report that systolic blood pressure generally rises with age until age 64, and then declines. The heart returns to its resting rate more slowly after exercise, and heart rates over 120/minute are poorly tolerated (p. 89).

The anterior chest is observed for any obvious deformities, lesions, or pulsations. The ball of the hand is used to first locate the point of maximum impulse (PMI) or the apex of the heart. This should be located at the fifth intercostal space in the left midclavicular line. Percussion is not generally performed in the physical assessment of the heart. However, this technique may be used to define the borders of an enlarged heart.

The large flat diaphragm of the stethoscope is first used to listen to the heart sounds. Beginning at the PMI, the stethoscope is gradually moved up the chest, to the left of the sternum. The first and second heart sounds (S_1 and S_2) are first identified. S_1 is the louder sound at the PMI. S_2 is the louder sound at the top of the heart. The sounds should be of equal intensity at Erb's point, or the third left intercostal space. The sounds are evaluated for rate, rhythm, and intensity. There should be no extra sounds, although a "splitting" of the S_2 is considered to be normal on inspiration. Identification and evaluation of heart sounds is dependent upon the skill and experience of the assessor. The physician must be notified if murmurs or extracardiac sounds are heard. Murmurs are best heard with the smaller bell of the stethoscope. The bell must be well sealed against the skin surface. Data from phonocardiographic studies show that murmurs are present in 60 percent or more of aging clients. The most common murmur is a soft systolic ejection murmur heard at the base of the heart (Malasanos, Barkauskas, Moss, & Stoltenberg-Allen, 1981, p. 628).

The blood pressure is taken in both arms, seated, standing, and lying. Serial blood pressures should be taken if there are known cardiovascular problems or if the person takes medication for high blood pressure. Bates (1983) states that variations of 10 mm Hg from arm to arm are considered normal (p. 185). The National High Blood Pressure Coordinating Committee (September, 1979) estimated that more than 40% of individuals over age 65 are hypertensive (Malasanos et al., 1981, p. 628).

The carotid arteries are gently palpated individually. The diaphragm of the stethoscope is gently placed on the carotid artery to determine the presence/absence of abnormal sounds called bruits, which are caused by impeded blood flow. The jugular veins are observed for distention, preferably with the head of the bed or examining table raised at a 45° angle. The peripheral pulses (radial, brachial, femoral, popliteal, dorsalis pedis, and posterior tibialis) are evaluated for the presence/absence, quality, and intensity. The apical pulse is compared with the radial pulse rate.

ABDOMEN

The principal age-related changes in the stomach, small intestine, and colon are decreased motility and peristalsis. There is a decrease in the production of gastrointestinal secretions, and a delay in emptying time of the stomach. There is also a decrease in the number of cells on the absorbing surfaces of the small intestine. The liver becomes smaller and there are decreases in weight and hepatic blood flow. Liver function declines with age. The gallbladder has a slower emptying time, and the bile becomes thicker and has less volume.

The usual order of inspection, palpation, auscultation, and percussion is altered in the assessment of the abdomen. Instead, the sequence is inspection, auscultation, percussion, and palpation. The abdomen is inspected for symmetry and abnormalities of contour which could indicate obstruction, hernia, or tumor. Arterial pulsations also may be noted. Any scars, striae, or dilated veins are also noted.

The diaphragm of the stethoscope is placed lightly on the abdomen. All quadrants are auscultated. Bowel sounds should be present throughout the abdomen. Absence of sound throughout the abdomen is a medical emergency. It is always suggested to listen for bowel sounds a minimum of 5 minutes.

The size of the liver and spleen and the location of the stomach can be determined by percussing the abdomen. Percussion is begun upward on the right side to identify the border of the liver. The sound elicited changes from tympany to dullness over the liver. The stomach is usually located slightly left of the midline in the area of the left rib cage. The spleen can be palpated in the area of the 10th rib on the left side.

Palpation of all four quadrants of the abdomen is done lightly with the fingertips. Light palpation is done to identify masses, tenderness, and location of abdominal organs. If the person complains of any pain or tenderness, palpation should not be done. The authors recommend that only light to moderate palpation be performed due to potential for injury occurring to underlying structures.

MUSCULOSKELETAL SYSTEM

The number of muscle cells and elastic tissue decreases with the aging process. The skeletal muscles atrophy, and strength and size decrease. Cartilage tissue thins and tends to yellow. The joints become less mobile. Changes occur in the vertebral column, which result in decreased height. Bone mass decreases and demineralizes, resulting in bones becoming brittle. The older client will have decreased muscle size as muscle mass declines with aging (Malasanos et al., 1981).

The person's gait is observed for limps, hemiparesis, and other abnormalities. The shoes should be observed for excessive wear on the heels, which can indicate a gait disturbance. The person's ability to sit and rise from a chair is also observed. The limbs are measured for equality of length and girth to establish baseline data. Muscle strength and integrity are assessed by having the person perform the following movements:

1. Squeeze the examiner's hands.
2. Shrug the shoulders against the force of the examiner's hands.
3. Flex the knees and push against the examiner's hands with the feet.

Range of motion test is also evaluated. The examiner does not perform the range-of-motion test, but asks the person to accomplish the above movements.

The hands are evaluated for the presence of Herberden's and Bouchard's nodes and Dupuytren's contractures. Herberden's nodes are hardened areas on the dorsal surfaces of the distal joints of the fingers. Bouchard's nodes are located at the proximal joints of the fingers. Both Herberden's and Bouchard's nodes suggest arthritis. Dupuytren's contractures involve nodular thickenings on the palm of the hand. The fingers may be pulled toward the palm and the person may be unable to completely extend the fingers. This contracture is most common among persons who are diabetic.

The joints are palpated for crepitus, which feels like "crackling" within the joint. Only light pressure should be used to avoid causing pain.

Some kyphosis or exaggeration of curves of the vertebral column will occur with aging. This is sometimes referred to as "dowager's hump."

NEUROLOGICAL SYSTEM

The brain declines in size and weight with advancing age. A nonfunctional substance called amyloid increases. Neurotransmitters decrease, resulting in the slowing of the reflexes. There is a decreased ability to respond to multiple stimuli. The number of neurons decreases, but the length of the dendrites increases (Podlone & Millikan, 1981, p. 115).

Intelligence and the ability to learn do not decrease, although more time may be required for processing information. Memory remains intact, although, according to Walker and Hertzog (1975, p. 160), short-term memory may decline with advancing age.

The neurological assessment may be initiated by observing the level of consciousness and general demeanor. A mental status examination should be performed. Emotional illness is estimated to be present in 20% of older adults and 40% in older adults with physical illness (Malasanos et al., 1981). Numerous tools of varying complexity have been devised for this assessment. The nurse is referred to *Confusion: Prevention and Care* by Wolanin and Phillips (1981) for a more complete discussion and description of evaluation tools.

The chief components of a brief mental status questionnaire (MSQ) are testing of recent and remote memory, orientation, calculation, consciousness, and graphic ability. The following questions can be asked:

1. (Nurse) My name is _____ .
2. What is your name?
3. Who is your doctor?
4. Do you know where you are?
5. How old are you?
6. When is your birthday?
7. Where do you live?
8. Who do you live with?
9. Do you remember what my name is?

Graphic ability can be assessed by asking the person to write his or her name. The ability to calculate can be assessed by the use of mathematical flash cards or playing cards. This asessment can also serve as a vision check.

The nurse should pay special attention to the person's speech; any unusual slowness, the lack of nouns in the speech, repetition of words or phrases, stuttering, or inappropriate responses should be noted.

The integrity of the cranial nerves (CN) may be assessed. However, the nurse must remember that the age-related changes can result in a slowing of the responses. To assess cranial nerve I, the olfactory nerve, the examiner holds a piece of scented material such as an alcohol swab, testing one nostril at a time while compressing the other nostril. Detection of the correct odor is a normal response; however, the sense of smell is diminished with aging.

Visual acuity and visual fields are tested when examining cranial nerve II, the optic nerve. A description of how to test visual acuity and visual fields may be found on pages 31–32. Assessment of the muscles of the eye (cranial nerves III, IV, VI—oculomotor, trochlear, and abducens) may be of little value because of age-related loss of convergence ability. Surgical procedures, such as cataract extractions performed on the eye, can also influence the appearance of the eye and reaction time.

The integrity of the trigeminal and facial nerves (cranial nerves V and VII) is tested by asking the person to frown, clench the teeth, show the teeth by raising the upper lip, tightly close the eyes, make chewing movements of the jaw, and puff the cheeks and smile.

The branch of the facial nerve that exits just anterior to the tragus of the ear can be gently tapped to elicit Chvostek's sign. A positive response is a facial tremor, and can indicate hypocalcemia.

The snout reflex of Wartenburg, if present, is indicative of diffuse cerebral dysfunction (Podlone & Millikan, 1981, p. 120). It is elicited by applying brief pressure to the lips. A positive response is a puckering movement of the lips.

The acoustic nerve, cranial nerve VIII, is tested as described on page 32. According to Eliopoulos (1984, p. 154), if the sense of smell is absent in both nostrils, the cause is not likely in the nervous system.

The integrity of the glossopharyngeal (IX) nerve is tested by touching the tonsillar area very lightly with a cotton-tipped applicator. The nerve is intact if the person gags. At the same time the integrity of the vagus (X) nerve can be evaluated by observing any uvular deviation. Cranial nerve (XI), the spinal accessory nerve, is tested by asking the person to shrug his or her shoulders. A lag of one side and inability to resist downward pressure of the examiner's hands on the shoulders is abnormal. The integrity of the hypoglossal (XII) nerve is assessed by asking the person to protrude the tongue while observing for any deviation.

Great care should be used when evaluating deep tendon reflexes (DTRs) to avoid causing injury or pain to joints that may be tender or arthritic. The Babinski sign may be elicited by lightly stroking the lateral aspect of the sole of the foot from the heel to the ball and across the ball. A positive response, which is indicative of upper motor neuron paralysis, is dorsiflexion and fanning of the toes. The older person will have decreased strength of reflexes but it should be possible to elicit all reflexes (Malasanos et al., 1981, p. 631).

A convenient method of evaluating sensation or lack of sensation in the various areas of the body is through the use of a tuning fork or small hand-held vibrator. The vibrating tuning fork, or another vibrating device, is placed on the various surfaces of the body and over the major joints. The person reports when vibration is perceived. This test may be performed first with the person's eyes open and then repeated with the person's eyes closed.

GENITOURINARY SYSTEM

The kidneys are primarily responsible for the regulation of fluid volume and soluble solids in the body. It is known that shifts in body composition occur with age. Water content decreases, while fat concentration increases. Kidneys decrease in size and lose the ability to concentrate urine, especially at night. There is reduced bladder capacity and loss of muscle tone. The bladder may fail to empty completely upon urination. Among males, there is a decline in the bactericidal secretions from the prostate (Judson, Novotony, McAnish, & Scott, 1981, p. 169).

Sexual desire, capabilities, and functioning remain intact throughout the life span in healthy adults. Among females, the menses and ovulation cease with menopause. The ovaries and uterus decrease in size. The vagina becomes thinner and less elastic, lubrication is decreased, and vaginal secretions become more alkaline.

Among males, spermatoza production continues throughout life, but the number and motility decrease. The size and firmness of the testes will decrease with aging (Bellack & Bamford, 1984, p. 533). The decline in reproductive function is more gradual among males than females. It takes longer for an older male to achieve an erection and reach a climax, and the amount of ejaculate is reduced.

Internal pelvic examination and Pap smear collection for the female and the prostatic exam of the male are generally done by the physician. The nurse is referred to Bates (1983) for a description of these procedures.

ENDOCRINE SYSTEM

Hormone secretion decreases with advancing age, which results in widespread effects in the body. In addition to lower levels of production, tissue response to hormones decreases. An example of the latter is a reduction in the ability of cells to utilize insulin, even though insulin levels are adequate. Sundwall, Rolando, and Thorn (1981, p. 142) report a normal decrease in glucose tolerance with aging. Changes also occur in the immune system, which result in slowing of repair of tissue damage. Production of antibodies and lymphocytes declines, causing increased susceptibility to disease. Further research should reveal more precise data regarding changes in the immune system associated with aging.

Many physiologic changes occur as a natural part of the aging process in all living things, from the smallest amoeba to man, the most sophisticated and cellularly differentiated organism. Humans have endeavored throughout history to define and describe what causes aging in cells, the basic unit of life. Many theories have been proposed, but as yet there is no clear-cut answer, although much promising research is in progress.

At the cellular level, the most outstanding age-related change is the accumulation of pigment called lipofuscin. This is a brownish substance commonly called "age pigment." The effect of this pigment on the body's physiology is not understood. The pigment does not accumulate in all tissues, but is commonly found in neural, muscle, liver, spleen, heart, adrenal, and pancreatic tissue (Denney, 1975, p. 204).

For physiological purposes, aging can be defined as the loss of function of cells or the inability of cells to replace themselves. Another definition of aging is the diminished ability to respond to stress. It is not completely clear which changes are the result of a disease process or which are in fact an inherent part of the normal aging process. Further study and research needs to be done to distinguish between the normal aging process and the pathological or disease-caused process. Does disease cause aging, or does aging cause disease? The answer to this question is not known.

A suggested physical assessment worksheet is provided on pp. 46–53.

PHYSICAL ASSESSMENT WORKSHEET

A. GENERAL SURVEY

Height: Weight (recent changes):

Vital signs: Blood pressure (sitting, standing, supine):

                    Temperature:
                    Heart rate:
                    Respirations:

General appearance:

B. INTEGUMENTARY SYSTEM

Color: Rashes:
Moisture:
Texture:
Temperature: Discoloration:
Turgor:

Hair:
  Thickness:
  Texture:
  Lubrication:

Scalp:
  Contour:
  Lesions:

Nail:
  Thickness:
  Circulation:

C. HEAD AND NECK

Head:
  Size:
  Shape:
  Contour:

Face:
   Temporal and masseter muscles (CN V, VII):
   Sinus area:
     Frontal:
     Paranasal:
     Maxillary:

Eyes:

   Visual acuity (CN II):

   Visual field:

   Extraocular movements (CN III,IV,VI):

   External eye structures:

   Pupils: Pupillary reflex (CN II):
           Direct and consensual:
           Pupillary accommodation:

   Internal eye structure:
         Red reflex:

Ears:
   External ear structure:

   Middle ear structure:
     Tympanic membrane:

   Hearing acuity (CN VIII):

     Rinne test:

     Weber test:

Nose:
   Patency:

   Olfactory sense (CN I):

   Asymmetry:

Inflammation:

Deformity:

Mucosa:
  Color:

  Lesions:

  Discharge:

  Swelling:

  Evidence of bleeding:

Septum:
  Deviation:

  Lesion:

  Superficial blood vessels:

Oral cavity:
  Color:

  Texture:

  Hydration:

  Contour:

  Lesions:

  Mouth odor:

Teeth: Dentures:
  Number:
  Status:

Palates and uvula (CN IX, X):

Tongue (CN XII):

Pharynx:
Infection, inflammation, lesions:

Neck:
General structure:

Trachea:

Thyroid:

Masses (determine size, shape, tenderness, consistency, and mobility):

Muscles (CN XI):

Shoulder shrug:

Lymph nodes:

D. LUNGS

A-P diameter:

Chest wall (anteriorly, posteriorly, laterally):
Contour:

Deformities:

Retraction:

Bulging of intercostal spaces:

Movement during respiration:

Percussion

Lung sounds:

Fremitus:

Diaphragmatic excursion: R._____cm
                                L._____cm

E. CARDIOVASCULAR

Pulses (rate and rhythm, amplitude —0 to 3 +):

Apical:

Radial:

Carotid pulse:

Brachial:

Femoral:

Popliteal:

Dorsal pedis:

Posterior tibial:

Jugular vein:

Heart sounds:

PMI:

F. BREASTS

Size:

Symmetry:

Color:

Retraction, flattening, contour:

Nipples:

Nodes:

G. ABDOMEN

Shape:

Symmetry:

Movement:

Umbilicus:

Bowel sounds:
   Intestinal motility:
   Vascular sounds:

Liver:
   Midclavicular liver span:

H. FEMALE REPRODUCTIVE

Discharge, itching, burning:

I. MALE REPRODUCTIVE

Discharge, itching, burning:

J. RECTUM

Hemmorrhoids:

K. MUSCULOSKELETAL

ROM:

Gait:

Posture:

Deformity:

Stiffness or instability of joints:

L. SPINE

Contour, position, motion:

M. FEET

Skin lesions:
  Callus(es):   Fissures between toes:

  Corn(s):   Redness:

  Edema(s):   Temperature:

Toenails:
  Thickened:
  Ingrown:
  Overgrown:

N. NEUROLOGICAL

Sensory:

  Pain:

  Tactile:

  Temperature:

  Vibration:

  Position change stimuli:

Motor function: Coordination:
  Upper extremities: Lower extremities:
  Romberg sign:

Cranial nerve summary (I-XII):

Reflexes (0-absent, 1-decreased, 2-normal, 3-increased, 4-spasticity):

Brachioradialis:

Biceps:

Triceps:

Abdominal scratch:

Patellar:

Achilles:

Plantar:

LEARNING CHECK

1. Wrinkling of the skin is caused by loss of _____ and of _____ tissue.

2. Hyperpigmentation is commonly called _____ _____ .

3. Generally, the organ system that undergoes the greatest age-related decline in function is the _____ system.

4. There are decreases in the _____ and tone of the muscles associated with respiration.

5. There are decreases in the number of _____ and dilatation of the _____ with age.

6. All of the age-related changes that occur in the respiratory system result in decreased _____ of tissues.

7. One millimeter for every year of age over 60 to age 90 should be subtracted from the _____ value of ABGs.

8. Heart muscle becomes _____ with age.

9. The most common murmur found at the base of the heart is _____ _____ _____ .

10. The heart _____ thicken and become more rigid.

11. Generally _____ blood pressure rises until age 64.

12. With aging, there is decreased _____ response to hormones as well as decreased hormone production.

13. Age-associated changes in the immune system include declines in the production of _____ .

14. The teeth become worn with age because of _____ .

15. The main change in the gastrointestinal tract is decreased _____ _____ .

16. The _____ decreases in size and weight.

17. The gallbladder has a slower _____ _____ .

18. Although color vision decreases, the _____ colors are perceived better by older persons.

19. In the ears, there is a decrease in the production of _____ with aging.
20. Muscles decline in _____ and _____ with aging.
21. There is thinning and yellowing of the _____ with advancing age.
22. _____ decreases due to changes in the vertebral column.
23. Bone mass decreases and _____ with aging.
24. Sexual _____ and _____ remain intact throughout the lifespan.
25. Lubrication of the vagina becomes more _____ with aging.
26. The functional decline in the reproductive system is more gradual in _____ than in _____ .
27. Water content _____ while body fat content _____ with age.
28. Kidneys lose the ability to _____ urine with advancing age.
29. There is reduced bladder _____ and loss of muscle tone, resulting in inability of the bladder to completely _____ .
30. Among males, the bactericidal secretions from the _____ gland decline.
31. A nonfunctional substance called _____ increases in the brain with aging.
32. Slowing of the reflexes is due to decreases in the amount of _____ .
33. The ability to learn and intelligence do not decline with aging, although _____ memory may decline.

REFERENCES

Armstrong, M., & Cleary, M. (1982). *Physiology of aging, part II*. Villanova, PA: ProScientia.

Bates, B. (1983). *A guide to physical assessment* (3rd ed.). Philadelphia: Lippincott.

Bellack, J., & Bamford, P. (1984). *Nursing assessment: A multidimensional approach*. Monterey, CA: Wadsworth Health Science Division.

Bennett, J., Creamer, H., & Fontana-Smith, D. (1981). Dentistry. In M. O'Hara-Devereaux, L. Andrus, & C. Scott (Eds.), *Eldercare*. New York: Grune and Stratton.

Carotenuto, R., & Bullock, J. (1980). *Physical assessment of the gerontologic client*. Philadelphia: Davis.

Denny, P. (1975). Cellular biology of aging. In D.S. Woodruff & J.E. Birren (Eds.), *Aging: Scientific perspectives and social issues* (p. 20). New York: Van Nostrand.

Eliopoulos, C. (1984). *Health assessment of the older adult*. Reading, MA: Addison-Wesley.

Interpreting arterial blood gases. (1980). *American Journal of Nursing*, 80(12), 2197–2201.

Judson, L., Novotony, T., McAnish, J., & Scott, J. (1981). Genitourinary system. In M. O'Hara-Devereaux, L. Andrus, & C. Scott (Eds.), *Eldercare* (p. 169). New York: Grune and Stratton.

Malasanos, L., Barkauskas, V., Moss, M., & Stoltenberg-Allen, K. (1981). *Health assessment*. St. Louis: Mosby.

Podlone, M., & Millikan, D. (1981). Neurology. In M. O'Hara-Devereaux, L. Andrus, & C. Scott (Eds.), *Eldercare*. New York: Grune and Stratton.

Sundwall, D., Rolando, J., & Thorne, G. (1981). Endocrine and metabolic. In M. O'Hara-Devereaux, L. Andrus, & C. Scott (Eds.). *Eldercare*. New York: Grune and Stratton.

Walker, J., & Hertzog, C. (1975). Aging, brain function, and behavior. In D.S. Woodruff & J. E. Birren (Eds.), *Scientific perspectives and social issues*. New York: Van Nostrand.

Wolanin, M.O., & Phillips, L. (1981). *Confusion: Prevention and care*. St. Louis: Mosby.

PART II

Actual or Potential Health Problems of Older Persons

The purposes of this part are to:
1. *Cite differences in the symptomatology of health problems frequently incurred by the elderly*
2. *Suggest possible nursing diagnoses relative to various actual or potential health problems of the elderly*
3. *Suggest certain nursing interventions appropriate for the nursing management of these health problems*

Introduction

The elderly are often afflicted with numerous health problems that make assessment difficult. Because of the "normal" physiologic changes outlined in the previous section, older persons, especially those who are debilitated, are more likely to develop diseases or health problems than persons of younger ages. Furthermore, acute illnesses may be manifested differently in older persons, and the onset may not be detected. For example, fever is not a frequent early symptom of respiratory infection in older persons, and many of the elderly experience heart attacks without chest pain. Older persons, as well as caregivers, may ignore "aches and pains" and perceive such discomforts as a normal or expected part of the aging process.

Additionally, older persons frequently take numerous medications that may mask or confound symptoms of disease or be the basis for some health problems. In the following chapters, various health problems and disease processes that commonly afflict the elderly are discussed.

3

Respiratory Problems

Common health problems of the respiratory system of the older adult can be related to characteristic changes that occur. The thorax becomes stiffer, lungs less elastic, and expansion of the rib cage more limited, resulting in lungs that are poorly aerated. As a result of structural changes, vital capacity decreases-as residual volume increases resulting in an alteration in the exchange of gases in the lungs. Common health problems of the older person include pneumonia, emphysema, and tuberculosis. The purpose of this chapter is to guide the nurse in careful analysis of the data obtained in order to allow the nurse to formulate valid nursing diagnoses with appropriate nursing interventions for clients with health problems of the respiratory system.

PNEUMONIA

Pneumonia is the inflammation of the lungs caused by bacteria, viruses, chemicals, or allergens. The elderly and debilitated are more susceptible to pneumonia due to declines in respiratory function, which include less effective coughing, and changes in the immune system. Fever and pleuritic pain are often absent; confusion and restlessness may be the only symptoms. Influenza and pneumonia are the fourth leading causes of death among older persons according to the Census Bureau (U.S. Department of Commerce, 1975).

Examples of Potential Nursing Diagnoses

1. Ineffective airway clearance due to tenacious secretions.
2. Impaired gas exchange due to ventilation–perfusion imbalance.
3. Alteration in nutrition (less than body requirements) due to loss of appetite, fatigue.
4. Decreased activity tolerance due to fatigue.
5. Sleep pattern disturbance due to coughing.
6. Alteration in comfort due to pleuritic pain.
7. Potential for impairment of skin integrity due to immobility.
8. Alteration in bowel elimination, constipation, due to immobility.

Potential Nursing Interventions

1–2. Improve airway clearance and gas exchange:
   a. Position in the semi- or high-Fowler's position if the person cannot assume or maintain the position for postural drainage.
   b. Splint the chest with small pillows or a bath blanket.
   c. Maximize coughing effort by teaching/assisting the person to take a deep breath, breathe again, and cough on the second exhalation.
   d. Maintain adequate humidity to prevent drying of secretions through the use of a continuous vaporizer. If a vaporizer is unavailable, vessels of water may be placed on room heating sources, or the person can be transported to a high humidity area, such as a shower room or bathroom.
   e. Auscultate the lung fields frequently for the presence of adventitious sounds and effectiveness of airway clearance.

f. Suction only when necessary to maintain patency of the airway. If possible, preoxygenate the person before suctioning. Do not apply suction when inserting the catheter. Do not suction longer than 15 seconds and allow sufficient time for the person to recover from the procedure.

Nursing Consideration: The suctioning procedure may damage airway tissues and can also induce anoxia. The procedure is often very frightening and uncomfortable for the patient. Secondary or nosocomial infection also frequently results from improper suctioning technique.

3. Maintain adequate nutrition for body requirements:
   a. Encourage fluid intake to at least three to four quarts a day, if tolerated and not contraindicated by other conditions such as congestive heart failure or renal impairment (Billings & Stokes, 1982).
   b. Monitor and record intake and output.
   c. Provide frequent small feedings rather than large meals at regular mealtimes and assist with eating if necessary.
   d. Administer or assist with oral hygiene at frequent intervals and keep a supply of ice chips and tissues at the bedside to prevent drying of mucous membranes.

4–5. Conserve body resources to increase activity tolerance and allow for adequate rest and sleep:
   a. Plan necessary procedures and activites; allow for the patient to rest after procedures/activities.
   b. Alter institutional schedule (e.g., bath time, meal time, medication time) to meet the needs of the resident.
   c. Omit unnecessary procedures/activities (e.g., shampooing) until resident is better able to tolerate activity.

6. Relieve discomfort due to pleuritic pain:
   a. Medicate as/if ordered before pain occurs.
   b. Splint chest and maximize coughing effort as described above (#1).
7. Implement skin care measures/protocols to prevent pressure sores:
   a. Change position every 2 hours and massage pressure points if skin is intact and redness blanches (Shannon, 1984).
   b. Use sheepskins, egg-crate mattresses, or other pressure-relieving devices when resident initially becomes bedfast or immobile.
8. Prevent constipation:
   a. Encourage fluid intake.
   b. Add bran, prune juice, or cranberry juice to diet.
   c. Position the person in most upright position possible for toileting; use toilet if the activity tolerance permits.

Nursing Consideration

The nurse should also monitor the health record to determine if the person has received influenza and pneumococcal vaccinations. If immunity has not been established, notify the physician or follow institutional protocols for immunization.

EMPHYSEMA

Emphysema occurs when the alveoli of the lungs are distended or ruptured. There is an accompanying loss of lung elasticity. The symptoms are slow in onset and resemble normal age-related changes in the respiratory system. Weakness, weight loss, and loss of appetite are common symptoms. Restlessness and dyspnea develop later in the disease.

Examples of Potential Nursing Diagnoses

Diagnostic statements include those lists in the "Pneumonia" discussion. "Anxiety, severe, related to ineffective breathing" and "Knowledge deficit, use of medication" are other nursing diagnoses to consider when planning the care of the person with emphysema.

Potential Nursing Interventions

1. Improve airway clearance and gas exchange:
   a. Teach breathing exercises, including "pursed-lip" breathing. Pursed-lip breathing is accomplished by having the person inhale slowly and deeply while the lips are "puckered-up" as if to whistle.
   b. Encourage coughing with short "huffs" rather than sustained coughing action.
   c. Administer and monitor oxygen therapy with a physician's order.
   Nursing Consideration: The flow rate of oxygen should never exceed 2–3 L/min to avoid overriding the brain's triggering mechanism of breathing. The nurse must be vigilant for signs of hypoxia, which include:
      1. Increased pulse rate
      2. Restlessness
      3. Flaring of the nostrils
      4. Intercostal and sternal retractions
      5. Disorientation

   Nasal hygiene should be administered frequently if oxygen is administered to prevent dryness of the nasal membranes. This procedure can be accomplished by encouraging the person to blow his nose, and cleansing the nasal membranes with a moistened applicator. A lubricant may be sparingly applied if the membranes are excessively dry.

2. Conserve body resources to increase activity tolerance and allow for adequate rest and sleep:
   a. Allow person to rest in the position of greatest comfort. The person with emphysema is often more comfortable in a chair, recliner, or in a high-Fowler's position in bed.
   b. Keep the room environment cool.
   c. Use an overbed table for the person to lean over while in bed or in a chair for support.
3. Reduce anxiety:
   a. Have an anxious or dyspneic person focus on the nurse's breathing pattern. Breathe slowly, deeply, using the pursed-lip technique.
   b. Relaxation training also may be helpful in relieving anxiety associated with inability to breathe effectively (Davis, Eshleman, & McKay, 1982).
4. Teach the correct use of hand-held medication nebulizers:
   a. It is necessary to have a physician's order for self-medication and medication at the bedside.
   b. Examine the package insert for precise instructions since variations can exist among products.
   c. The use of such devices must be monitored because of potential overuse of such medicine.

TUBERCULOSIS

Tuberculosis is the infectious disease of the lungs caused by the tubercle bacillus, *Mycobacterium tuberculosis*. Blake (1981, p. 420) states that the incidence of this disease is greatest among the older age group. This is probably due to immunological changes that occur with aging. Although fever and night sweats are common symptoms of this disease, these symptoms do not occur frequently among the elderly. Anorexia, weakness, and hemoptysis are common symptoms. Although screening for tuberculosis should be performed for all persons entering a long-term care facility, persons who are known positive reactors to the skin-testing agent should not be retested since intense local reactions may occur. According to Carroll (1984) positive diagnosis of tuberculosis is made by sputum smear and culture.

Examples of Potential Nursing Diagnoses

Diagnostic statements include those listed in the pneumonia and emphysema sections. "Social isolation" should be considered as a nursing diagnosis if isolation measures are utilized to reduce contagion.

Potential Nursing Interventions

Interventions include those listed in the previous sections. Other interventions may include the following:

1. Maintenance of nutritional status with high protein, high carbohydrate diet.
2. Implementation of isolation measures, if indicated, and if confirmed by appropriate diagnostic studies. Teach the person to cover the mouth with tissue when coughing, and to correctly dispose of tissues.
3. Allaying possible fear and stigma of affected person among other residents, family, and staff through teaching.

LEARNING CHECK

1. _____ is not a frequent symptom of respiratory infection in older persons.
2. The older person should be assisted to cough by _____ the chest with pillows.
3. Drying of secretions can be prevented through the use of a _____ .
4. One of the most important considerations in caring for

persons with respiratory problems is to allow enough time for _____ .

5. It is frequently helpful to teach persons with emphysema _____ breathing.

6. _____ must be administered with extra care to an older person who has emphysema.

4

Cardiovascular Problems

According to Jacobs (1981, p. 34), cardiovascular diseases account for the greatest number of deaths among older persons. Angina, myocardial infarction, and hypertension are the most common cardiovascular diseases among older adults. Other common cardiovascular diseases of older adults include peripheral vascular disease, atherosclerosis, and anemia. Signs of cardiovascular health problems are cardiac enlargement, abnormal cardiac sounds, fine moist rales, and distended neck veins. Symptoms of cardiovascular health problems are dyspnea on exertion, orthopnea, tachycardia, anorexia, and nausea/vomiting. The development of signs/symptoms may be very insidious, and they are often not noticed by older persons or caregivers. Older persons who have cardiovascular disease usually complain of having cold hands and feet. Nursing interventions usually consist of reducing cardiac workload, effective use of digitalis and diuretic drugs, and reducing sodium and water retention through diet. The purpose of this chapter is to guide the nurse in developing nursing diagnoses and nursing interventions with common health problems of the cardiovascular system.

MYOCARDIAL INFARCTION

Heart attack or myocardial infarction, which is the occlusion of a coronary artery or its branches, may be asymptomatic in older persons. Tissue damage and death of heart muscle always result from a myocardial infarction. Acute chest pain is often absent. Pain, if any, may be in the shoulder or jaw, and vague indigestion may be present. Symptoms may progress rapidly to shock and cardiac arrest.

Potential Nursing Diagnoses

1. Alteration in comfort due to pain
2. Alteration in tissue perfusion due to erratic cardiac filling
3. Fear of impending death

Nursing Priorities

1. Assess physical status and monitor vital signs.
2. Obtain emergency medical assistance.
3. Institute emergency lifesaving measures if necessary.

Potential Nursing Interventions

1. Relief of pain, discomfort:
   a. Place person in position of greatest comfort.
   b. Loosen any constricting clothing.
   c. Note location, quality, onset, and duration of pain.
   d. Take a subjective measurement of pain: Have the person rate intensity of pain on a scale of 1 to 10 with 10 being the most severe pain.
2. Improve tissue perfusion:
   a. Administer oxygen.
   b. Monitor pulse and blood pressure continuously; auscultate heart sounds.
   c. Observe for mottling of the skin, paleness, cyanosis, diaphoresis, tightening of the shoulder girdle, neck vein distention.
3. Relieve fear, anxiety:
   a. Keep the environment as calm and quiet as possible.
   b. Stay with the afflicted person at all times; have others summon assistance, supplies.
   c. Remove unnecessary persons from the area.

CONGESTIVE HEART FAILURE

Congestive heart failure is that condition in which cardiac output is inadequate to meet the body's needs. Eliopoulos (1979, p. 143) states that mental confusion, insomnia, wandering about during the night, and peripheral and presacral edema may be signs of this condition. A hacking cough, distended neck veins, and rapid weight gain may also be noted. An S_3 (third heart sound) is often heard in congestive heart failure.

Potential Nursing Diagnoses

1. Decreased cardiac output due to increased cardiac workload
2. Alteration in comfort due to chest pain, dyspnea
3. Alteration in fluid volume, more than body requirements, due to ineffective cardiac pumping
4. Potential for fluid volume deficit due to use of diuretics
5. Potential for impairment of skin integrity due to immobility and stasis

Potential Nursing Interventions

1. Decrease the workload of the heart to improve cardiovascular status:
   a. Monitor vital signs; take apical pulse rate.
   b. Assess heart and lung sounds. An S_3 (third heart sound) is often heard in congestive heart failure.
   c. Maintain bedrest during acute phase; record vital signs after activity.
   d. When changing an occupied bed, change bed linens from the head of the bed down, instead of from side-to-side, to decrease work load of the heart.
   e. Plan and space activities to avoid fatigue.
   f. Assist with eating if necessary.

2. Relieve chest pain, discomfort:
   a. Place person in semi- or high-Fowler's position.
   b. Provide overbed table for support if orthopnea is present.

3–4. Maintain adequate/proper fluid balance:
   a. Monitor and record intake and output.
   b. Weigh daily at same time with the same scale.
   c. Observe for edema; measure and record abdominal or peripheral girth.
   d. If fluids are restricted, give frequent mouth care; offer ice chips, hard candy, chewing gum (unless contraindicated). Ice chips must be counted in the fluid allotment.
   e. Observe for signs of potassium depletion if diuretic therapy is used. Signs and symptoms include malaise, muscle weakness, faint heart sounds, silent bowel sounds, "gassy" abdominal distention (Kintzel, 1977, p. 503).

5. Maintain skin integrity:
   a. Use sheepskins, egg-crate mattress, or other special pads.
   b. Change position of the bedfast person frequently.
   c. Massage bony prominences, pressure points, if tissues blanch well and are intact.

HYPERTENSION

Age-associated blood pressure changes were discussed in the preceding section. Older persons who have high blood pressure frequently awaken with a dull headache, have impaired memory, and may have epistaxis.

Potential Nursing Diagnoses

1. Alteration in tissue perfusion due to increased cardiac workload

2. Alteration in comfort, headache
3. Potential for injury, falls, associated with weakness and/or dizziness

Potential Nursing Interventions

1. Decrease the myocardial workload:
   a. Monitor the blood pressure in both arms with the person seated, lying, and standing.
   b. Encourage rest periods throughout the day and following activity.
   c. Teach relaxation techniques. The nurse is referred to *The Relaxation and Stress Reduction Workbook* by Davis, Eshleman, and McKay (1982) for a comprehensive discussion of teaching relaxation techniques.
2. Relieve discomfort, headache:
   a. Eliminate or decrease agents that may cause vasoconstriction(e.g., caffeine, nicotine). Ice water may be safely given without danger of vasoconstriction (Howser, 1976).
   b. Limit physical activity.
3. Prevent injury, falls:
   a. Teach the person to rise slowly from the bed or chair and to sit on the edge of the bed for a few moments before ambulating.
   b. Instruct the person to sit or lie down and to summon assistance if dizziness occurs.
   c. Keep the bed in the low position.

Nursing Considerations

1. Blood pressure needs to be closely monitored if hypertension medication is prescribed, since the person may sustain a lowering of the blood pressure that is too low for body needs.
2. To control or slow epistaxis, bend the head slightly forward, apply an ice pack to the back of the neck, and apply

pressure for at least 10 minutes to the lower part of the nose by gently pinching the nostrils together.

ANGINA

Angina, or chest pain due to decreased oxygenation of the myocardium, may be less severe in older adults than in younger age groups. Symptoms may include vague discomfort, which often occurs after a meal.

Potential Nursing Diagnoses

1. Alteration in comfort due to chest pain
2. Potential for injury, falls, due to weakness
3. Potential for impairment of skin integrity due to application of medication "patches" or irritating ointments

Potential Nursing Interventions

1. Relieve chest pain:
   a. Administer medication as ordered.
   b. Decrease physical activity.
   c. Provide small, frequent meals to decrease cardiac workload.
2. Prevent potential injury, falls:
   a. Instruct person to sit or lie down at first perception of pain, chest tightness, or discomfort.
   b. Encourage person to rest after meals, activity.
   c. If a form of nitroglycerin is prescribed for relief of symptoms, the person should recline for 15 to 20 minutes after use of the medication to prevent dizziness.
3. Maintain skin integrity:
   a. Rotate and record ointment or patch application sites
   b. Carefully cleanse area after the patch is removed. If the

skin is extremely sensitive, the route of administration should be changed.
c. Record and report reddened, irritated areas to the physician.

Nursing Considerations

1. Caution must be used to avoid self-absorption of the medication through the fingers when applying cutaneous vasodilating agents.
2. Patches must not be applied to any scar tissue on the person's body.

LENEGRE'S DISEASE

Carotenuto and Bullock (1980) describe Lenegre's disease as a process in which microscopic lesions develop in both bundle branches of the conduction system of the heart. The coronary arteries or myocardium are not involved. Symptoms include fainting, loss of consciousness, and seizures (p. 95).

Potential Nursing Diagnoses

1. Alteration in cardiac output, decreased heart rate
2. Potential for injury, falls

Potential Nursing Interventions

1. Decrease cardiac workload:
   a. Monitor vital signs, especially after activity.
   b. Investigate medication and dietary intake to identify possible predisposing factors.
2. Prevent injuries, falls:
   a. Teach the person to recline or sit down upon onset of symptoms.
   b. Implement seizure precautions, if indicated.

Nursing Considerations

1. Have *oral airway* at resident's bedside and at *predetermined* location at nursing station and on medicine cart.
2. Have suction equipment "ready to go."
3. Pad siderails only if indicated.
4. Have predetermined means of communication established for staff to respond to seizure situations (e.g., "Code Yellow").
5. Never attempt to force the victim's jaws open during a seizure; do not restrain the limbs.
6. Remove victim's dentures only if dentures are loose and occluding the airway.
7. If it is necessary to insert an airway, ease the oral airway between the teeth when the victim's jaws begin to relax *IF* the teeth are biting down on the tongue or *IF* the airway is impaired.
8. Note and document the time, duration, loss of consciousness, and body parts involved.

Other Considerations

Digitalis preparations are frequently prescribed for older persons with heart problems. However, due to normal as well as disease-induced changes in the body, toxic levels of this drug may result. Symptoms of digitalis toxicity include weakness, vertigo, and visual disturbances, including greenish-yellow vision, bad dreams, and hallucinations. The pulse must be monitored before administration of this type of drug. If the pulse rate is below 60 beats per minute, digitalis preparations should be withheld. When a drug is withheld, the reason must be documented. Whenever possible, the person receiving digitalis preparations should be instructed to monitor and record his or her own pulse rate.

ANEMIAS

Older persons often become anemic for a variety of reasons. They may be anemic because of chronic insidious blood loss, such as bleeding from hemorrhoids or gastrointestinal bleeding associated with long-term aspirin use. Older persons may be anemic because of poor nutritional or dietary practices. Ill-fitting dentures and dental and periodontal problems may prevent the older person from eating properly. Additionally, older persons with impaired mobility and/or vision may be unable to accomplish shopping and cooking tasks. Limited finances also may have reduced the amount of foods with high nutrient density that can be purchased. It is also reported by Moehrlin, Wolanin, and Burnside (1981, p. 330) that older persons who live alone may fail to eat properly because of loneliness, depression, and dislike of eating alone.

Persons with anemia complain of weakness, anorexia, hypersensitivity to cold, and other vague complaints that may be attributed to "old age." As the anemia advances, mental confusion may occur. A thorough medical examination as well as dietary history should always be accomplished.

Iron Deficiency Anemia

Iron deficiency is the most common cause of anemia in older persons. This condition can be medically corrected with iron supplements according to Walraven, Malik, and Cyr (1981, p. 236). Although iron is better absorbed when the stomach is empty, these supplements should be given initially with meals to improve tolerance.

Potential Nursing Diagnosis

1. Alteration in nutrition, less than body requirements, related to inadequate dietary intake of iron

Potential Nursing Intervention

1. Maintain adequate nutrition and iron intake
   a. Assess the condition of the mouth, teeth, dentures
   b. Encourage dietary intake of foods high in iron (meats, soybean flour, beans, etc.).
   c. Initially administer oral iron preparation with meals; if no side effects occur, administer preparation when the stomach is empty.

Pernicious Anemia

Pernicious anemia is also common among older persons and is due to lack of a specific factor in the gastric secretions necessary for the absorption of vitamin B_{12} according to Walraven et al. (1981, p. 239). Persons with pernicious anemia usually complain of a sore tongue (which appears reddened and ridged), weakness, and numbing and tingling of the extremities. These persons may not be able to perceive vibration and may have a loss of the Achilles' tendon reflex. Pernicious anemia is medically treated with Vitamin B_{12} injections.

Potential Nursing Diagnoses

1. Alteration in nutrition, less than body requirements, due to glossitis
2. Sensory perceptual alteration, coldness related to alteration in temperature
3. Potential for injury, falls, bruises, associated with increased risk of falling due to weakness

Potential Nursing Interventions

1. Maintain adequate nutrition, body weight:
   a. Provide oral hygiene before and after meals with a very soft brush or cotton ball.
   b. Avoid foods that are very hot or highly seasoned.

2. Keep person warm, avoid chilling. (See also specific interventions listed in Chapter 10, "Hypothyroidism.")
3. Prevent injuries:
   a. Observe for changes in gait.
   b. Assist with ambulation if necessary.
   c. Teach the person to rise, move slowly.
   d. Have necessary objects within reach of person.

LEARNING CHECK

1. An older person may sustain a myocardial infarction
   without _____ _____ .
2. The disorder involving microscopic lesions of the bundle
   branches of the heart is _____ _____ .
3. A dull headache upon awakening and confusion may
   indicate _____ .
4. Digitalis preparations should not be given if the pulse
   rate is below _____ .
5. An older person may experience fainting or dizziness
   after taking _____ .
6. Night wandering may indicate _____ _____ .
7. The most common cause of anemia among older persons
   is _____ _____ .
8. Iron preparations are best absorbed when the stomach is
   _____ .
9. Pernicious anemia is related to the malabsorption of
   _____ _____ .
10. Persons with pernicious anemia usually complain of
    _____ _____ .

5

Urinary Problems and Problems of the Reproductive Organs

The most common health problem of the older person is incontinence. The healthy older person tends to pass urine more frequently with an increased degree of urgency. Other problems include urinary tract infections, neurogenic disorders, and prostratic hypertrophy among males. Control of urine is vital to the older person for both social and hygienic considerations. The purpose of this chapter is to provide information to guide the nurse in formulating and developing nursing diagnoses and the suggested nursing interventions for the client with health problems of the genitourinary system.

URINARY PROBLEMS

Incontinence

Incontinence, the involuntary loss of urine, is the chief urinary problem of older persons. Eliopoulos (1979, p. 229) states that this condition may be due to multiple causes, including weakness of the muscles, inability of the kidneys to concentrate urine, neurological problems, certain medications, infections, and mechanical causes such as calculi and prostatic enlargement. However, the most common cause of urinary incontinence in the elderly is fecal impaction. Additional causes of incontinence can include dehydration, poor vision, which prevents locating the toilet, and alteration in mobility, which prevents the person from reaching the toilet.

Potential Nursing Diagnoses

1. Alteration in urinary elimination, incontinence
2. Self-care deficit related to inability to toilet self
3. Potential for infection due to wetness, perineal irritation
4. Disturbance in self-concept related to incontinence
5. Knowledge deficit, urinary control measures

Potential Nursing Interventions

1. Assess the cause of incontinence:
   a. Observe and record episodes of incontinence to determine a pattern. A convenient method, suggested by Autry, Lawson, and Holliday (1984), uses self-adhesive "dots" to record incontinence. The dots are applied to a time log to indicate when incontinence occurs, when the person is dry, and when toileting is done. The log should be maintained for at least 1 to 2 weeks for accuracy and to determine a pattern.
   b. Check for fecal impaction by digital examination. Gently percuss the abdomen for bladder distention.
   c. Inspect external genitalia for redness, irritation, discharge. Wash the perineal area gently with mild soap and water, and rinse and dry thoroughly after the episode of incontinence. Apply olive or mineral oil to the area to provide lubrication if necessary.
   d. Collect a urine sample. Note the urine for color, cloudiness, purulence, and odor. Perform a "dipstick" test for sugar, ketones, blood, and protein. Obtain an order for a complete urinalysis and culture and sensitivity.
   e. Review medications for potential side effects related to incontinence. Hypnotics, antianxiety agents, and sedatives may contribute to incontinence.

f. Assess the environment. Determine if the toilet is too high or too low. If the seat is too low, use a "high-rise" toilet seat; provide a commode if the seat is too high. Assess the lighting in the bathroom. The area should be well lit but glare free. If the toilet facilities are distant from the resident's room, provide a commode. Provide privacy.

g. Assess hydration. Maintain fluid intake of 1500 to 2000 cc per day, unless contraindicated by other health problems. Provide fluids that acidify the urine such as cranberry and prune juice. Avoid caffeinated beverages, which may promote diuresis and urgency.

2. Assist with toileting to maintain dryness:
   a. Use the toilet or bedside commode unless impossible.
   b. Design a realistic toileting schedule, and involve the person in schedule planning. Toilet before and after meals, planned activities, bedtime.
   c. Facilitate voiding by running water when urination is desired. Have the person blow into a glass of water with a straw to initiate urination.
   d. After assessing the record of incontinence, toilet the person before usual time of episode.
   e. Assess "cues" for need to void, if a communication deficit exists. Such cues may include restlessness, agitation, or touching the lower abdominal or perineal area.

3. Provide personal hygiene to prevent infection:
   a. Cleanse perineal area as described in item 1c.
   b. Use soft absorbent bathroom tissue or facial tissue after voiding. Teach the person to blot the perineal area dry and to wash hands after voiding. Ascertain the effectiveness of the person's efforts of perineal hygiene.

4. Maintain the person's positive self-image:
   a. Praise all efforts to maintain dryness.
   b. Involve the person in planning and implementing the control program.
   c. Never scold or reprimand if incontinence occurs.

5. Teach measures to promote urine control:
   a. Determine the length of time necessary to reach the bathroom or commode. Teach the person to allow adequate time to reach the toilet.
   b. Teach methods, such as Kegel's exercises, to increase pelvic muscle strength. Instruct the person to practice tightening the anus as if attempting to hold back stool. If possible, instruct the person to alternately start and stop the stream of urine when voiding to increase meatal control.

Bladder Infections

Armstrong and Cleary (1982, p. 4) state that bladder infections are the most common cause of fever in older persons. Common symptoms include burning, urgency, and abdominal pain. As a urinary tract infection progresses, the person may retain urine and develop incontinence and/or hematuria. Acute infections may be medically managed with antibiotic or antiseptics; however, chronic infections tend to be less responsive to drug therapy and often recur when the medication is stopped.

Potential Nursing Diagnoses

1. Alteration in urinary elimination related to frequency, urgency
2. Alteration in comfort due to abdominal pain, burning

Potential Nursing Interventions

1. Restore the normal voiding pattern:
   a. Increase fluid intake unless contraindicated by other health problems.
   b. Provide beverages that acidify the urine, including cranberry and prune juice.
   c. Provide commode if the person has mobility problems or if the bathroom is distant.

  d. Use disposable incontinence products if necessary to avoid embarrassment and wetness.
2. Relieve pain related to infection:
  a. Apply moist compresses to perineal area.
  b. Carefully cleanse perineum after voiding and bowel movements.
  c. If the person is able to use the bathtub, soak in a tub filled to the level of the umbilicus. Use warm sitz baths.
  d. Assess the person's temperature at the same time every day. Be alert for slight rises in the temperature, which may indicate fever in older individuals.

Benign Prostatic Hypertrophy

Benign prostatic hypertrophy, or enlargement of the prostate gland, is present among the majority of older men. Initially, symptoms of frequency, nocturia, decreased urinary force, dribbling, and inability to initiate the stream occur. As the condition progresses, there is urinary retention, pain in the flank and/or lower abdomen, and hematuria. If unrecognized or uncorrected, kidney damage (hydronephrosis) may occur. Surgical intervention is necessary to correct this condition.

Potential Nursing Diagnoses

1. Alteration in urinary elimination related to inability to empty the bladder
2. Sleep pattern disturbance due to nocturia
3. Alteration in comfort, pain, due to bladder distention

Potential Nursing Interventions

1. Relieve urinary retention:
  a. Record intake and output.
  b. Gently palpate and percuss suprapubic area to identify bladder distention.
  c. Push fluids during the day to promote kidney and bladder flushing.

d. Catheterize, with physician's order, if necessary.

e. Assist or instruct the person to stand when voiding.

2. Promote sleep/rest:

a. Restrict fluid intake 1 to 1½ hours before bedtime.

b. Check for bladder emptying and/or distention at bedtime.

c. Use disposable incontinence products during the night if leakage is a problem.

3. Relieve pain due to bladder distention (see also measures cited in item 1 and in the "Bladder Infection" section of this chapter).

Indwelling Catheters

It is never desirable for older persons to have permanent indwelling catheters. Carroll (1984) states that infections and inflammation of the urinary system occur without fail with the use of catheters. However, at times, the use of an indwelling catheter cannot be avoided. Meticulous perineal and meatal care must be performed for the older person, especially after bowel movements. Indwelling catheters should be secured to the abdomens of males to facilitate drainage and prevent pulling on the catheter. When caring for uncircumcised males, the caregiver must be certain to replace the foreskin over the glans penis. Painful, marked swelling of the penis, which may lead to tissue necrosis, may occur if this is not done.

Potential Nursing Diagnoses

1. Potential for infection due to indwelling catheter
2. Alteration in urinary elimination related to catheterization

Potential Nursing Interventions

1. Prevent urinary tract infection:

a. Provide perineal care.

b. Maintain a closed drainage system. Obtain samples

only through aspiration ports. Do not use catheter plugs.
c. Do not routinely irrigate catheters unless absolutely necessary. Instead, encourage oral fluids.
d. Do not routinely change indwelling catheters. Change only when the patency is impaired.
2. Attempt to restore normal voiding pattern by discontinuing the catheter.

Nursing Considerations

Disagreement in the literature exists regarding the precise procedure for bladder retraining before catheter removal. Catheter removal should be carefully planned. The person should be involved in this procedure.

1. Begin bladder training by clamping the catheter to determine if the person can perceive bladder fullness. Do not clamp for longer than 2 hours to avoid potential overdistention.
2. Assess for distention when the catheter is clamped.
3. Observe the person closely for bladder distention and the need to void. Nursing measures described in the section on incontinence may also be employed.

PROBLEMS WITH REPRODUCTIVE ORGANS

Many older women believe that gynecological examinations are not necessary after the childbearing age, menopause, or hysterectomy. Although the incidence of cervical cancer declines with age, examinations must be continued to detect other types of malignancies as well as benign conditions of the reproductive system.

Vaginitis

Vaginitis is a common problem of older women. Symptoms include vaginal discharge, soreness, and itching. Confused or noncommunicative persons may be restless and scratch the genital area.

Potential Nursing Diagnoses

1. Alteration in comfort: pain and itching
2. Potential for impairment of skin and mucous membrane integrity due to irritation
3. Knowledge deficit, need for gynecological examinations

Potential Nursing Interventions

1. Relieve pain and itching:
   a. Maintain perineal hygiene. Wash the area with mild soap and water, rinse well, and dry thoroughly. Apply prescribed ointments or lubricate area with olive or mineral oil.
   b. Apply moist compresses to affected area.
   c. If vaginal suppositories or ointments are prescribed, instill medication while the person is lying in bed to achieve the best effect. The side-lying position may also be used.
2. Maintain integrity of perineal tissues:
   a. Institute hygienic measures described above.
   b. Provide sitz baths, avoiding excessively warm solutions that may damage fragile tissue.
   c. If douching is ordered, select the proper size of douche tip to avoid tissue injury. Monitor the temperature of douche solutions. Be sure that prepackaged solutions are not too cold.
3. Health teaching, need for gynecological examination
   a. Explain the need for procedure or examination.
   b. Explain the procedure or examination.

Prolapse

Prolapse of the uterus or other pelvic part may occur among older women as a result of the stretching and tearing of muscles during childbirth and muscle weakness associated with aging. Signs and symptoms may include visible protrusion of parts, low back pain, and pelvic pulling.

Potential Nursing Diagnoses and Interventions

Nursing diagnoses and interventions include those cited in the previous section. Additional interventions are:

1. Observe and record the time, frequency, and appearance of the prolapsed part.
2. Protect the prolapsed part with sterile vaseline gauze and padding.
3. If possible, have the person lie down and assume the knee-chest position to reduce the prolapse.

LEARNING CHECK

1. _____ is the chief urinary problem of older persons.
2. Nursing interventions to deal with incontinence are determined by the _____ .
3. The most common cause of fever in older persons is _____ _____ .
4. The majority of older men have some degree of _____ _____ _____ .
5. Care must be taken to replace the _____ of uncircumcised males after hygienic measures.
6. Restlessness and itching may be a symptom of _____ in older women.
7. As a result of stretching of muscles during childbirth, _____ _____ may occur with aging.

6

Gastrointestinal Problems

Common health problems of the gastrointestinal system consist of problems of ingestion, digestion, and elimination that are necessary to support growth and maintain metabolism. Common health problems of the older person include diverticulosis and gallbladder disease. Also included are hemorrhoids, fecal impaction, hernias, and periodontal disease. The purpose of this chapter is to provide the nurse with information about identifying potential or actual nursing diagnoses and nursing interventions for clients with common health problems of the gastrointestinal system.

XEROSTOMIA

The condition of the mouth and teeth is a primary consideration in sound nutrition. Periodontal disease can predispose the aged to systemic infection. Xerostomia, or dryness of the oral mucosa, may result from decreased production of saliva and/or use of medications such as anticholinergics and antidepressants. Good oral hygiene is especially important for the aged who have losses in the number of taste buds.

Potential Nursing Diagnosis

1. Potential for impairment of oral mucosa

Potential Nursing Interventions

1. Maintain integrity of the teeth and oral mucosa:
   a. Brush the teeth and tongue with a soft toothbrush or foam brush after each meal. Gentle flossing should also be done.
   b. Correct xerostomia by the application of a mixture suggested by Ettinger (1982) which consists of 20 cc of methylcellulose (Metamucil®), 10 cc of glycerine, and 60cc of water.

HIATAL HERNIA

Hiatal hernia is the protrusion of the proximal portion of the stomach into the thoracic cavity through the diaphragm. Morgan, Thomas, and Schuster (1981, p. 203) state that hiatal hernia occurs in as many as 67% of persons over age 60. Signs and symptoms of this condition include heartburn, belching, and vomiting after meals, especially when reclining or bending forward. This condition is aggravated by increased abdominal pressure.

Potential Nursing Diagnoses

1. Alteration in comfort due to pain
2. Alteration in nutrition, less than body requirements, due to inability or reluctance to eat and retain food

Potential Nursing Interventions

1. Relieve discomfort:
   a. Position patient upright in a recliner or in semi-Fowler's position after meals. Blocks may be positioned under the head of the bed to achieve elevation.
   b. Do not feed the person in bed unless sitting up is impossible or contraindicated.

    c. Avoid increasing intra-abdominal pressure by encouraging resident to wear loose clothing and restricting the use of girdles and corsets. Prevent constipation.
2. Maintain weight and adequate nutrition:
    a. Provide several small meals rather than three large meals.
    b. Supplement meals with high protein feedings.
    c. Instruct the person to eat slowly and maintain an upright position for 30 minutes after each meal (Billings & Stokes, 1982, p. 977).

DIVERTICULOSIS

Diverticuli, or multiple pouches of the intestinal mucosa of the large bowel, are very common among older persons. Bowel contents can accumulate in these pouches, causing inflammation known as diverticulitis. Pain usually occurs in the left lower quadrant. Constipation is often present, and nausea and vomiting can also occur. Hospitalization is frequently necessary during an acute attack.

Potential Nursing Diagnoses

1. Alteration in comfort, pain
2. Alteration in bowel elimination, constipation
3. Alteration in fluid balance, less than body requirements, due to nausea
4. Alteration in nutrition, less than body requirements, due to loss of appetite, nausea

Potential Nursing Interventions

1. Relieve abdominal pain:
    a. Assess abdomen for presence, absence, or hyperactivity of bowel sounds, pain, tenderness, or distention; record findings.

    b. Apply ice pack to the abdomen, if pain is severe, while awaiting physician's orders.
2. Prevent constipation:
    a. Encourage high fiber, high residue diet, fluids.
    b. Administer suppository every 2 days if the person has not had a bowel movement.
    c. Avoid the use of enemas to prevent irritation of the bowel.
3. Maintain adequate hydration:
    a. Assess mucous membranes for moisture; gently palpate eyeballs for "mushiness" (a sign of dehydration.)
    b. Record intake and output if urine output is <30 cc/hr.
4. Maintain weight, adequate nutrition:
    a. Provide a high fiber diet, supplemental feedings.
    b. Weigh every 2 to 4 weeks.

GALLBLADDER DISEASE

Gallbladder disease is the most common cause of severe abdominal pain among elders according to Morgan and associates (1981, p. 202). Fever is present, and pain is in the right upper quadrant. Jaundice may be present. Surgery, if indicated, is often postponed until the person's condition improves. Persons with gallbladder disease often report intolerance to certain foods. Pork, fatty foods, and popcorn are frequently cited as causing distress.

Potential Nursing Diagnoses

Diagnostic statements include those cited in the hiatal hernia and diverticulitis sections of this chapter. Additional diagnostic statements include the following:

1. Alteration in nutrition, less than body requirements, due to food intolerance

2. Potential for impairment of skin integrity due to accumulation of bile salts in blood, which causes pruritus

Potential Nursing Interventions

1. Maintain adequate nutrition:
   a. Assess for food intolerances.
   b. Substitute other foods that do not cause distress to provide adequate nutrition.
2. Maintain skin integrity:
   a. Observe sclera for yellowing.
   b. Shake urine and observe for frothing (if bile is present, the urine will foam).
   c. Do not use soap on the skin; keep the skin lubricated with an oil-based product.

HEMORRHOIDS

Hemorrhoids, while usually asymptomatic, may cause health problems for elders. The person may complain of intense anal itching and pain. Streaks of bright red blood may appear in the stool, on toilet paper, or undergarments. Hemorrhoids are aggravated by constipation, sitting for long periods of time, and by frequent digital examinations of the rectum. Constipation frequently occurs because the person may attempt to ignore the urge to defecate to avoid pain.

Potential Nursing Diagnoses

1. Alteration in comfort, pain
2. Alteration in bowel elimination, constipation

Potential Nursing Interventions

1. Relieve anal/rectal pain:
   a. Observe and record episodes of blood in the stool.
   b. Provide flotation pad when resident is sitting.

   c. Wash anal area carefully with soft cloth or facial tissue, and dry with soft cloth.

   d. Use ice packs initially on anal area to reduce edema; use warm compresses or sitz bath after initial 15 to 20 minutes of ice application to soothe and to promote circulation.

   e. Avoid performing digital rectal examinations to avoid aggravating hemorrhoidal pain.

2. Prevent constipation:
(see section on constipation/fecal impaction in this chapter)

CONSTIPATION/FECAL IMPACTION

Constipation and fecal impaction are frequent problems of older persons. Inactivity, immobility, less dietary bulk, and laxative abuse add to the development of these conditions. Measures should be taken to prevent the conditions.

Potential Nursing Diagnoses

1. Alteration in bowel elimination, constipation/fecal impaction
2. Knowledge deficit related to diet, resulting in constipation

Potential Nursing Interventions

1. Prevent constipation:
   a. Record bowel elimination to determine a cycle or pattern.
   b. Maintain adequate fluid intake.
   c. Provide high fiber diet; obtain order for stool softener if indicated.
   d. Determine what practice the person uses to achieve bowel movement, and implement, if acceptable.

  e. Administer suppository every two days if a bowel movement has not occurred.
2. Relieve fecal impaction:
  a. Assess for impaction by gently performing digital examination of the rectum. Explain the procedure carefully. Position the person on the left side. Gently insert the well-lubricated, gloved index finger through the anus anteriorly, and gently palpate for feces. A topical anesthetic ointment, such as Xylocaine®, may be applied before the procedure to relieve discomfort.
  b. Administer a stool softening (oil retention) enema, if ordered. Hydrogen peroxide, if ordered, can also be instilled rectally to break up impacted stool (Mager-O'Conner, 1984).
  c. If the above measures fail, the impaction may be removed manually. Two gloved and lubricated fingers can be inserted to break large, hard stool into smaller pieces that can be evacuated. Manual removal of stool must be done very slowly and gently. The procedure must be stopped and the physician consulted if the person complains of severe pain or if bleeding occurs.
  d. A small packaged enema may be administered to complete evacuation after manual removal of stool.

Nursing Considerations

Large-volume enemas should not be given to elderly persons. According to Mager-O'Conner (1984) shock can result from the sudden distention of the large bowel.

LEARNING CHECK

1. _____ , or excessively dry oral mucosa, results from decreased saliva production.

2. Heartburn and belching after meals are frequent symptoms of _____ .

3. A _____ _____ diet is helpful in the prevention of constipation.

4. The most common cause of severe abdominal pain among older persons is _____ .

5. The best method of dealing with constipation is _____ .

7

Musculoskeletal Problems

Osteoporosis and osteoarthritis are common health problems that effect changes in balance, posture, and mobility in older adults. Some of the most common health problems of older persons are related to changes that occur in muscles, bones, and joints. The older person is at high risk for falls and fractures. There is too often a fine line that distinguishes pathology from normal aging changes. The purpose of this chapter is to provide information about musculoskeletal problems of the older person and to assist the nurse in developing nursing diagnoses with possible nursing interventions for the client.

OSTEOPOROSIS

Osteoporosis is the most common bone disease afflicting older persons. Jacobs (1981, p. 31) describes osteoporosis as characterized by demineralization of the bone, resulting in decreases in bone mass and density. Immobilization accelerates this condition. Older persons often believe that pain, which frequently occurs in the vertebrae and lower limbs, is due to "rheumatism." The exact cause of osteoporosis is not known, but its development is related to the dietary intake of calcium, protein, and phosphate; metabolism of Vitamin D;

and deficits of estrogen. Compression fractures of the vertebrae are a common complication of osteoporosis.

Potential Nursing Diagnoses

1. Impaired physical mobility due to stiffness
2. Alteration in comfort, pain
3. Potential for physical injury, fracture
4. Knowledge deficit related to dietary intake of calcium, protein, and phosphate

Potential Nursing Interventions

1. Improve mobility by improving muscle strength:
   a. Obtain physical therapy consultation.
   b. Encourage sedentary exercises, such as arm extensions, arm curls, stationary rocking, other range of motion exercises.
   c. Avoid prolonged immobility.
2. Relieve pain:
   a. Take a careful history to determine precipitating factors such as certain activities, temperature variations, which may result in pain.
   b. Medicate, if ordered, before onset of pain.
3. Prevent falls, fractures:
   a. Encourage the proper use of canes, walkers if gait is unsteady.
   b. Instruct person to rise from chairs, bed slowly.
   c. Check footwear; well-fitting, low-heeled shoes should be worn.
   d. Use great care and gentleness when moving or exercising a person with osteoporosis to avoid injury.
4. Instruct about foods that are high in calcium, protein, and phosphate.
   a. Obtain dietary consultation.
   b. Encourage selection of foods with necessary nutrients.

Nursing Consideration

Height loss accompanies the development of osteoporosis due to the gradual vertebral collapse. Richards (1982) recommends assessing the amount of spinal compression by having the person raise the arms sideways to shoulder level. The distance from the longest fingertip of one hand to the longest fingertip of the other hand is measured. In nondiseased persons this measurement is the same as the height. When vertebral compression due to osteoporosis has occurred, the height is less than the fingertips measurement.

OSTEOARTHRITIS

Osteoarthritis is the gradual thinning of joint cartilage. Symptoms include aching, stiffness, and limited motion of joints. The knee is the joint most frequently affected by this disease. Rossman (1981, p. 39) states that characteristic nodules, or thickenings, known as Heberden's nodes, often appear at the distal joints of the fingers. While these nodes are disfiguring, they usually are not disabling. The appearance of these nodes helps differentiate osteoarthritis from rheumatoid arthritis. Additionally, inflammation is usually absent in osteoarthritis.

Medical management of this condition usually involves a combination of medication, physical therapy, and exercise. Persons with osteoarthritis should be cautioned not to "overdo"; many persons with this problem experience pain following unusual activity.

Potential Nursing Diagnoses

1. Alteration in comfort, pain
2. Impaired physical mobility due to joint stiffness
3. Decreased activity tolerance due to immobility and pain

Potential Nursing Interventions

1. Relieve arthritic pain:
    a. Determine what method(s) the afflicted person uses to relieve pain and implement, if acceptable.
    b. Obtain medication history, including home remedies, to determine what medication provides the best relief.
    c. Apply moist heat to the affected areas if warmth relieves the pain.
    d. Use wool or sheepskin protectors on the affected joints to provide warmth and protection.
    e. Evaluate effectiveness of pain relief measures.
2. Improve physical immobility associated with joint stiffness:
    a. Obtain physical therapy consultation, if indicated.
    b. Maintain proper body alignment; instruct the person about proper body mechanics.
    c. Maintain and promote an exercise program, including range-of-motion and isometric exercises.
    d. Encourage the use of canes, walkers, for gait stability and safety.
3. Improve activity tolerance, conserve strength:
    a. Determine which activities (ADLs, therapeutic, social) are most painful or difficult for the person to accomplish.
    b. Medicate, if indicated, prior to planned activity times.
    c. Plan sequence of activities to conserve body resources.

RHEUMATOID ARTHRITIS

Rheumatoid arthritis involves inflammatory changes in the synovial membrane resulting in destruction of joint cartilage and deformities. Symptoms are extremely painful and swollen joints, especially in the morning; fever; fatigue; and malaise. Medical treatment is directed at the relief of inflamma-tion and pain. The exercise/therapy/activity plan must be carefully designed by a multidisciplinary team involving the physician, nurse, physical therapist, occupational therapist, and the afflicted person. Persons with rheumatoid arthritis can frequently benefit from the use of assistive devices, such as specially designed utensils, to foster self care.

Potential Nursing Diagnoses

Diagnostic statements include those listed in the os-teoarthritis section of this chapter.

Potential Nursing Interventions

Nursing interventions include those cited in the os-teoarthritis section of this chapter.

Nursing Considerations

During exacerbations of this disease, it is essential to rest the affected body part(s). Splinting is used to protect the affected part(s) from further injury and to prevent joint contractures.

The nurse must also be cognizant of various side effects of medications prescribed for the relief of symptoms, and close-ly monitor the afflicted person for the development of unto-ward reactions. Aspirin is frequently prescribed for relief of pain and inflammation. Long-term use of aspirin has been implicated in gastrointestinal bleeding and iron deficiency anemia.

HIP FRACTURES

According to Keene and Anderson (1982), as many as 45% of women 75 and older sustain hip fractures. Hip fractures may be due to many causes, including transient ischemic attacks, rapid drop in blood pressure, osteoporosis, and others. The caregiver should always be concerned with the cause of the fracture. Occasionally older persons who sustain fractured hips do not complain of pain, so the nurse should look for gait disturbances. On the other hand, intense pain that radiates to other muscle groups may be present. The affected hip is externally rotated, causing a spasm of the quadriceps muscle.

Potential Nursing Diagnoses

1. Alteration in comfort due to pain
2. Impaired physical mobility due to interruption of bone integrity
3. Potential for impairment of skin integrity
4. Potential for joint contractures

Potential Nursing Interventions

1. Relieve pain:
   a. Medicate as ordered.
   b. Apply ice to fracture site.
   c. Immobilize the affected hip with splints, sandbags, trochanter rolls.
2. Care following surgery depends upon the type of surgical correction performed. Ambulation is resumed as soon as possible.
3. Prevent joint contractures:
   a. Maintain functional alignment in bed.
   b. Implement and teach range-of-motion exercises.
4. Prevent pressure areas and decubiti:
   a. Institute special skin protocols.
   b. Use special mattress to avoid pressure.

LEARNING CHECK

1. Osteoporosis is characterized by _____ of the bones.
2. Joint inflammation is not usually associated with _____ .

right side of the brain results in paralysis of the left side of the body. There may also be memory deficits, impulsive behavior, and spatial–perceptual deficits. Damage to the left side of the brain results in paralysis of the right side and slow, disorganized behavior. Aphasia often results when the damage is on the left side of the brain. The aphasia may be receptive, that is, the brain of the affected person may not be able to process what the person reads, hears, or sees; or the aphasia may be expressive, that is, the person may be able to comprehend what is heard, seen, or read, but cannot form the words to respond to the stimuli. Aphasia may also be mixed, both receptive and expressive. This impairment is called conduction aphasia.

Visual problems, known as hemianopsia, also frequently occur with stroke. Right-sided paralysis, or hemiplegia, may be accompanied by the inability to see right of center in the visual field. Left hemiplegia may be accompanied by the inability to see left of center in the visual field. Depression and withdrawal, due to multiple physical changes and losses, may also follow a CVA.

Rehabilitation efforts must begin as soon as possible after the cerebrovascular accident occurs. Intense nursing efforts are necessary.

Potential Nursing Diagnoses

1. Alteration in cerebral tissue perfusion related to compromised blood flow
2. Ineffective airway clearance due to diminished cough reflex
3. Potential for fluid volume deficit due to inability to swallow
4. Alteration in nutrition, less than body requirements, due to inability to eat/drink
5. Alteration in bowel elmination, constipation, due to immobility, dietary changes

6. Alteration in urinary elimination due to immobility, fluid balance changes
7. Impaired physical mobility (specify deficit—e.g., related to right/left hemiplegia)
8. Potential for joint contractures due to immobility
9. Impaired communication, verbal and/or written
10. Potential for impairment of skin integrity due to immobility
11. Sensory-perceptual deficit, impaired vision
12. Body image disturbance due to loss of function and sensory neglect
13. Self-care deficit (specify)

Potential Nursing Interventions

1. Monitor neurological status to ascertain changes in homeostasis:
    a. Monitor and document vital signs (B/P, TPR); monitor femoral, popliteal, and pedal pulses.
    b. Monitor and document pupil size, pupillary reaction response to stimuli, presence/absence speech, orientation to person, place.
    c. Monitor and record intake and output.
2. Facilitate coughing effort and airway clearance:
    a. Assess patency of airway; auscultate chest for adventitous sounds.
    b. Maintain adequate humidity to prevent drying of secretions.
    c. Position person to maximize coughing effort, airway clearance.
    d. Suction only if necessary.
3. Maintain adequate hydration:
    a. Assess mucous membranes for moisture; gently palpate eyeballs for "mushiness" (sign of dehydration).
    b. Record intake and output.

    c. Assess integrity of gag reflex by gently touching the uvula with a cotton-tipped applicator. The open mouth can be stabilized by inserting the index finger on the middle of the lower tongue and applying mild pressure to the tissue.

    d. If the gag reflex is intact, the ability to swallow can be tested by instilling a small amount of fluid into the back of the mouth and instructing the person to swallow.

4. Maintain adequate nutrition:

    a. Assess the person's ability to swallow (see above).

    b. Seat the person upright if possible.

    c. Offer chewable rather than semisoft or pureed foods. Chewing seems to enhance the swallowing reflex (Sahs, Hartman, & Aronsen, 1976, p. 167).

    d. Check for proper denture fit, if applicable. If the person's dentures do not fit properly, the chewing and swallowing efforts will be better without the dentures.

    e. Stimulate the swallowing reflex by having the person suck briefly on an ice cube prior to eating. Immediately after the sucking, lightly stroke around the mouth three times with another ice cube. Using ice, then lightly stroke three times from both earlobes to the corners of the mouth. Following this stroking, use ice to stroke three times from the front of the ears along the jawbone to the center of the chin. Finally, apply the ice to the sternal notch for not more than three seconds. After the icing procedure, repeat the same procedure with a sable brush or a vibrating brush designed for this purpose (Williams, McDonald, Daggett, Schut, & Buckwalter, 1983).

    f. Place the food within the person's field of vision, and prepare the food within the field of vision

    g. Place the food in the unaffected side of the person's

mouth. Place a mirror in front of the person to teach correct placement of food in the mouth as suggested by Sahs et al. (1976, p. 167).

h. Provide privacy when feeding efforts are begun. Do not feed the person in a congregate dining room until the person has gained confidence in the ability to swallow.

i. Use specially designed utensils, or encase the handles of spoons and forks in foam to facilitate the grasp of the utensils.

5. Prevent constipation:
   (see Chapter 5, "Constipation/ Fecal Impaction" section)

6. Prevent urinary incontinence and retention:
   (see Chapter 6, "Incontinence" section)

7. Maintain optimal physical mobility:
   a. Assess and document extent of paralysis immediately and at regular intervals.
   b. Immediately begin passive range-of-motion exercises of all extremities at least twice a day.
   c. Splint, protect affected limbs.
   d. Pronate the person twice a day.
   e. Maintain functional alignment in bed.

8. Prevent joint contractures:
   a. Begin passive range-of-motion exercises immediately.
   b. Prevent shoulder contractures by supporting the arms with pillows or bath blankets when the person is in bed. As activity progresses, the affected arm should be supported in an appropriate sling.
   c. Use hard cones rather than soft materials to prevent contractures of the hand. Soft objects tend to promote flexion of the hand among stroke victims (Farber, 1982, p. 152).
   d. Use trochanter rolls and sandbags to prevent hip rotation.

e. Do not use footboards to prevent footdrop. The pressure of the footboard stimulates plantar flexion and causes pressure on the ball of the foot (Farber, 1982, p. 258). Footdrop is best prevented by pronation twice a day and by allowing the feet to extend over the end of the mattress.

9. Establish and maintain communication:
   a. Determine the native language of the affected person. Aphasic persons may begin verbal efforts with the native language.
   b. Talk directly to the person, using short, specific phrases and maintaining eye contact.
   c. Encourage the person to sing familiar rhymes/ditties to aid in communication. Persons with aphasia may be able to communicate by singing, even though speech is impaired (Rosenzweig & Leiman, 1982, p. 652).
   d. Use communication aids, such as velcro boards and pictures indicating basic needs and electronic speech equipment.

10. Prevent skin breakdown
    (see interventions listed in Chapter 11, "Skin Disorders")

11. Modify the environment to compensate for visual losses:
    a. Assess the scope of impairment (hemianopsia, diplopia) through visual assessment. This may be accomplished by asking the person to point to pictures on a printed page.
    b. Position the person (and the bed) so that persons and activities in the room are perceived in the intact field of vision. For example, if the person has a deficit in the right field of vision, position the bed so the left eye is used to view the room.
    c. Teach *all* staff and visitors to approach the person from the visually intact side.
    d. Patch the affected eye if diplopia exists.

12. Increase and facilitate the person's awareness of the para-
    lyzed limb/side:
    a. Teach the person to use the unaffected limb to move
       the affected part. For example, put the "good" leg
       under the paralyzed leg to facilitate position changes,
       transfer from the bed to a chair, and similar move-
       ments.
    b. Encourage exercises in which the limbs cross the mid-
       plane of the body, such as swinging the arms from
       side to side. The person can use the "good" arm to
       move the affected arm.
    c. Teach the person to gauge space and distance by over-
       estimating the size of doorways, length of halls, and
       distance to chair seats.

PARKINSON'S DISEASE

Parkinson's disease is a disorder of body movement characterized by four major symptoms:

1. Bradykinesia, or slowing of movement
2. The loss of postural reflexes
3. A "pill-rolling" tremor at rest
4. Muscle rigidity

Muscle rigidity, according to Podlone and Millikan (1981, p.
125), causes the greatest physical impairment. Other signs of
this disease are a mask-like facial expression, a festinating or
tripod gait, speech difficulties, and problems related to the
autonomic nervous system, including drooling, sweating,
urinary retention, constipation, and postural hypotension.
    The underlying cause of this disease is dysfunction of the
basal ganglia within the brain. These collections of nerve
cells and supporting tissues are the centers of motor coordi-

nation. A neurotransmitter called dopamine is manufactured by specialized pigmented cells called the substantia nigra, which is located in the basal ganglia. There are losses of these pigmented cells and depletion of the amount of dopamine in Parkinson's disease.

The principal medical treatment of this disease involves drugs to increase the level of dopamine and control tremor, such as levodopa and combinations of this drug. Persons receiving levodopa should be observed for development of a side effect known as tardive dyskinesia. Signs of this condition include a protruding tongue, bizarre facial and lip movements, and abnormal movements of the lower extremities. The development of tardive dyskinesia results more often from length of treatment than dosage level. Other side effects of levodopa are nausea, vomiting, anorexia, urinary retention, and orthostatic hypotension. Sexual arousal sometimes occurs from the use of this drug, according to Rosal-Greif (1982).

The long-term use of phenothiazines can also produce symptoms of parkinsonism and tardive dyskinesia. Symptoms usually disappear after the drug is discontinued.

Potential Nursing Diagnoses

1. Impaired physical mobility related to bradykinesia and muscle rigidity
2. Impaired verbal communication due to weakness of muscles associated with speech production
3. Alteration in nutrition, less than body requirements, due to difficulty in swallowing
4. Potential for infection, pneumonia, due to weakness of chest muscles
5. Alteration in urinary elimination, incontinence
6. Alteration in bowel elimination, constipation

7. Potential for impairment of skin integrity due to immobility
8. Disturbance in self-concept related to physical losses

Potential Nursing Interventions

1. Maintain/improve mobility:
   a. Carefully assess afflicted person to determine levels of mobility and reassess at periodic intervals.
   b. Teach the person to set the feet down heels first when walking and to increase the width of the stride.
   c. Teach the person to swing the arms when walking to improve balance.
   d. Encourage practicing "marching" to music.
   e. If "freezing" occurs when the person is walking, have the person "unfreeze" by raising the arms or trying to step backwards.
   f. Teach the person to rise from a chair by placing the feet apart and pushing against the arms of the chair.
   g. Encourage practicing fine motor function by picking up coins or marbles, typing.
   h. Perform or teach the afflicted person to perform range-of-motion exercises twice a day.
2. Improve and/or maintain verbal communication:
   a. Arrange for a speech pathologist/therapist, if necessary.
   b. Teach the person to take a breath before initiating speech and to speak when breathing out.
   c. Encourage the person to practice speech by repeating "nonsense" syllables, reading aloud, or singing.
3. Maintain adequate nutrition:
   a. Provide the person's with meals/trays first to compensate for slowness in eating in a congregate setting.
   b. Use specially designed utensils to facilitate grasp.
   c. See other interventions listed in this chapter under "Cerebrovascular Accident."
4. Prevent respiratory infection:
   (see interventions listed in Chapter 3, "Respiratory")

5. Prevent urinary retention, incontinence:
   (see interventions listed in Chapter 5, "Incontinence")
6. Prevent constipation:
   (see interventions listed in Chapter 6, "Constipation/Fecal Impaction")
7. Maintain skin integrity; prevent skin breakdown:
   (see interventions listed in Chapter 11, "Skin Disorders")
8. Increase self-esteem:
   a. Allow client to vent thoughts and feelings.
   b. Request referral to a psychosocial counselor.
   c. Inform client about benefits of medication.
   d. Encourage discussions of reflecting on past successes.
   e. Provide positive reinforcement about intact physical abilities.

ORGANIC BRAIN DISEASES

When an older person suddenly becomes confused or has a personality change, it should be regarded as an emergency. Diagnostic tests should be undertaken to determine the cause. Confusion is never a normal or expected part of aging. Organic brain diseases are the most debilitating of all ailments associated with aging in terms of human loss. Organic brain disease, while frequently listed in records as the medical diagnosis, is imprecise and may preclude adequate nursing assessment and interventions. These health problems are better classified as acute and chronic brain syndromes of a specific type. Acute and chronic brain syndromes are classified by times of onset.

Acute Brain Syndrome

Acute brain syndrome has a rapid onset. Symptoms include misidentification of persons, restlessness, night wandering, and visual hallucinations. Wolanin and Phillips (1981) suggest that acute brain syndrome may be caused by hypoxia, due to various anemias, cardiovascular/circulatory and respiratory problems; drugs; trauma; metabolic disorders, including thyroid and liver diseases, hypoglycemia/hyperglycemia, hypocalcemia/hypercalcemia; infections; hypothermia/hyperthermia; malnutrition and fluid/ electrolyte imbalances; and depression. Acute brain syndrome is medically treatable and recovery can be complete if quickly recognized, assessed, and treated.

Potential Nursing Diagnosis

1–2. Sensory–perceptual alteration related to change in homeostasis

Potential Nursing Interventions

1. Assess source/origin of confusion:
   a. Establish communication; use direct eye contact and touch; check vital signs.
   b. Perform mental status questionnaire; determine if the person knows his or her name, where he or she is; name of the physician; when his or her birthday is; whether he or she can perform purposeful activity (e.g., hand a nearby object to the nurse).
   c. Orient the person if errors are made in the mental status questionnaire.
   d. Investigate hallucinations/areas of confusion for potential validity.
   e. Perform neurological, respiratory, and cardiovascular assessment.
   f. Check for hypoglycemia/hyperglycemia; if possible, evaluate blood sugar with chemical strip analysis.
   g. Evaluate recent history for changes in medication, including discontinued medication; relocations; recent losses; changes in the environment.
   h. Notify the physician of person's condition.

2. Implement reality orientation measures to reduce/resolve confusion:
   a. Acknowledge the reality of the hallucination to the person. For example, in the case of a visual hallucination, state, "I know the spiders are very frightening to you, but I am unable to see them."
   b. Inform the person of caregiver's name, place, date, what has happened.
   c. Avoid the use of restraints unless necessary for the person's safety.
   d. Avoid overmedication if sedation and/or tranquilizers are prescribed.
   e. Maintain a quiet, calm environment; reduce unnecessary noise.

Chronic Brain Syndrome

Chronic brain diseases have a gradual onset. The hallmark of chronic brain disease is dementia. Dementia is chiefly characterized by intellectual deterioration, disorganization of the personality, and the progressive inability to carry out activities of daily living. Chronic brain diseases include multi-infarct dementia, Pick's disease, Huntington's chorea, Creutzfeldt-Jakob disease, and Alzheimer's disease.

Multi-infarct dementia probably accounts for about 20% of the chronic brain disorders and is due to diffuse cerebral arteriosclerosis. Symptoms are related to the amount and location of the damage to the cortex.

Pick's disease, Huntington's chorea, and Creutzfeldt-Jakob disease are relatively rare dementias. In Pick's disease the Pick cells located in the frontal portion of the cerebral cortex balloon and swell. The progress of this disease is usually rapid. Symptoms and signs are similar to Alzheimer's disease according to Podlone and Millikan (1981, p. 118). Huntington's chorea is characterized by manic mood changes and bizzare choreiform movements. Creutzfeldt-Jakob disease is caused by a slow growing virus that destroys cerebral tissue.

Mace and Rabins (1981) state that Alzheimer's disease (senile dementia, Alzheimer's type) is the most prevalent dementia among older persons. The underlying pathology of this disease is the development of neurofibrillary tangles and the accumulation of a plaque-like substance in the cerebral cortex that prevents the normal transmission/reception of stimuli. The exact cause of Alzheimer's disease is unknown, but there is an associated decrease in a neurotransmitter known as choline acetyltransferase in the brain. No specific diagnostic test exists for this disease. Medical diagnosis is made by ruling out other medical problems.

According to Prillaman and Junk (1984) Alzheimer's disease is generally characterized by four stages. The first stage is very insidious and generally lasts 2 to 4 years. Symptoms of this stage include progressive forgetfulness, deterioration of short-term memory, and progressive inability to do simple arithmetic. The person usually does not require admission to a long term care facility during this stage.

The second stage is characterized by more pronounced forgetfulness. The person does not initiate normal routines and may forget to perform usual hygiene. The speech becomes progressively slower and devoid of nouns. Disorientation to time and to day and night also is frequent in this stage. The person often becomes suspicious of persons around him or her, and frequently voices unfounded complaints of neglect or abuse. The course of this stage is variable; the person may remain in this stage for years or may progress rapidly into the third stage.

The third stage is characterized by the development of more pronounced signs and symptoms. The affected person develops aphasia, agnosia (the inability to attach meaning to sensory impressions), and apraxia (the inability to carry out purposeful movement). The "mirror sign," the inability to recognize oneself in the mirror, is noted, and the person may not recognize family or other loved ones. Catastrophic reactions, uncontrolled behavior frequently manifested by striking out and abusive language, may also occur in this stage. The person may also exhibit a great appetite but lose weight.

The fourth and final stage is characterized by even more pronounced deterioration. The person becomes incontinent, has marked weight loss, and has little or no response to stimuli. The person may also experience visual hallucinations and seizures.

Nursing diagnosis and interventions depend upon the stage of the illness. The nursing assessment and history provide the basis for planning the nursing care. Priorities include the following:

1. Determine a method of communicating; determine what words the person uses for voiding, bowel elimination, pain, hunger, thirst. Determine if the person speaks more than one language.
2. Determine if the person recognizes self and loved ones.
3. Determine what special senses are intact. A convenient method of assessing sight, hearing, motor control, and the ability to follow directions is the game SIMON™. This is a small electronic table game that produces four various sounds and four different colors in a random sequence. The participant is asked to repeat the color/sound sequence presented by the device by depressing the appropriate illuminated color section.
4. Determine what activities of daily living the person is able/unable to perform for himself/herself.

Potential Nursing Diagnoses

1. Alteration in thought processes related to inability to communicate
2. Memory deficit associated with person, time, and place

  3. Diversional activity related to inactivity
  4. Sleep pattern disturbance due to not sleeping at night
  5. Potential for physical injury due to impaired judgment
  6. Alteration in nutrition, less than body requirements due to inability to eat
  7. Potential for fluid volume deficit due to inability to recognize thirst
  8. Alteration in bowel elimination, constipation related to toileting deficit
  9. Alteration in urinary elimination, incontinence
 10. Potential for violence related to impaired judgment

Potential Nursing Interventions

  1. Establish communication to reduce undesirable behavior (specify):
     a. Stand directly in front of the person when communicating.
     b. Institute eye contact.
     c. Use touch when talking to the person.
     d. Use simple, short phrases.
     e. Do not argue with the person if argumentative; distract him or her with another activity.
     f. Stroke the person's face lightly upward and backward if he or she is noisy or disruptive.
  2. Implement measures to maintain orientation (specify): (Example: To assist person in remembering where his or her room is):
     a. Provide name sign on bed.
     b. Place familiar objects, picture, or color on door of room.
     c. Repeat information frequently throughout the day.
  3. Implement activity program consistent with the person's ability:
     a. Walk the person (outside, if possible) every day.

    b. Involve in reminiscence; begin with era of Great Depression (if appropriate for age).

    c. Have the person sort and identify old photos from the family.

4. Modify activites to encourage sleeping at night:

    a. Plan activities early in the day/afternoon.

    b. Reduce activities after supper. (Note: Physical activity results in fatigue, which increases confusion.)

    c. Do not restrain the person in bed unless absolutely necessary for safety.

    d. Draw privacy curtain, reduce lighting to give "night time" clues.

5. Reduce potential for injury through modification of environment:

    a. Remove or tape privacy locks in the room.

    b. Keep bell in place on the person's door.

    c. The person should wear an identification band stating "Memory impaired."

    d. Remove mirrors, glassware, and all unnecessary objects from the person's room.

6. Provide adequate nutrition to maintain specified weight:

    a. Feed or provide tray first.

    b. Present one food at a time at meal.

    c. Offer snacks at specified time.

    d. Remove unnecessary silverware, dishes from tray.

7. Maintain adequate hydration:

    a. Serve or provide glass of fluid every 2–3 hours.

    b. Specify beverage with meals.

    c. Measure and record intake.

8. Prevent constipation:

    a. Maintain bowel record.

    b. Provide high fiber foods; add bran to cereals.

    c. See other measures listed in Chapter 6, "Constipation/Fecal Impaction."

9. Implement measures to prevent incontinence:

    a. Place identification sign on bathroom door; color code all bathroom doors.

    b. See other interventions listed in Chapter 5, "Incontinence."

10. Reduce occurrence of catastrophic reactions:

    a. Observe for restlessness; restrict group activites if the person is restless or agitated.

    b. Stop and distract the person and remove to a quiet area if control is lost.

NORMAL PRESSURE HYDROCEPHALUS

Normal pressure hydrocephalus (NPH) can be classified as an acute or chronic brain syndrome. According to Podlone and Millikan (1981, p. 118), this condition is characterized by dilatation of the ventricles of the brain, stasis of the cerebral spinal fluid, and normal spinal fluid pressure. Persons with this condition develop a scissors-like gate, sudden incontinence, and confusion. Normal pressure hydrocephalus can be diagnosed medically by CAT scan and is treatable by surgical shunting. Early detection is the key to prevention of a chronic irreversible brain syndrome.

Nursing Diagnoses and Nursing Interventions

Please see nursing diagnoses and nursing interventions listed for acute and chronic brain syndrome in this chapter.

LEARNING CHECK

1. Parkinson's disease is characterized by a _____ tremor in the hands.

2. In Parkinson's disease the greatest physical impairment is due to _____ _____ .

3. Persons who receive levodopa for long periods of time may develop _____ _____ .

4. Recovery from TIA usually occurs within _____ .
5. Organic brain diseases are best classified as _____ and _____ .
6. _____ is most prevalent organic brain disease, or chronic dementia.
7. _____ is the third leading cause of death in the aged.
8. Signs and symptoms of stroke that may last a few minutes or hours are called _____ .
9. The severity of stroke depends upon _____ and _____.
10. Damage to the right side of the brain results in paralysis of the _____ _____ of the body.
11. The aphasia is called _____ _____ when the affected person is not able to process what he/she reads, hears, or sees.

9

Health Problems Associated with Vision and Hearing

Perception is based on the functional ability of the elderly person's senses that influences behavior. Sensory changes occur gradually with aging. The purpose of this chapter is to provide the nurse with information to assist in developing nursing diagnoses and nursing interventions of the older person's sensory problems resulting from sensory changes and the promotion of use of remaining sensory functions.

VISION

Taisch, Taisch, and Metz (1981, p. 268) state that glaucoma is the most serious eye disease of older persons. If untreated, total blindness will occur. A gradual loss of peripheral vision is an initial symptom. Later symptoms include pain in the eye(s) and the appearance of halos around lights.

Cataracts are caused by opacification and degenerative changes of the lens of the eye. Initially, there is often a marked improvement in the ability to read without glasses, but this is followed by blurred and dimmed vision. Several methods of surgical removal of cataracts are available. After surgery contact lenses are sometimes used for vision. There are also various types of contact lenses. The nurse must be aware of the various types of contact lenses and of the proper removal technique and cleaning procedures required for care.

Potential Nursing Diagnosis

1. Sensory-perceptual alteration related to decline in vision

Potential Nursing Interventions

1. Plan, organize environment and personal space to accomodate visual loss:
   a. Plan placement of the person's personal effects, water pitchers, and other significant objects with the person who has impaired vision, and do not alter the placement.
   b. At mealtimes place the food in a "clockwise" fashion and inform the person where the food is located.
   c. Place the visually impaired person's hand on the caregiver's upper arm and have the caregiver walk beside and slightly ahead of the person when guiding the person down halls or stairs.
   d. Always explain exactly what is to happen, or what is about to be done to the visually impaired person.
   e. Always knock on the door and identify yourself before entering the room and/or personal space; also inform the person when leaving the room.

HEARING

Hearing loss (presbycusis) is common among older persons; however, hearing impairment is not an expected consequence of aging. Hearing loss must be evaluated through audiometric testing. Additionally, older persons often develop impacted cerumen in the ears, which interferes with hearing and can lead to infection.

Potential Nursing Diagnosis

1. Sensory perceptual alteration related to hearing loss

Potential Nursing Interventions

1. Facilitate communication:
   a. Always face the hearing-impaired person and speak slowly with a low-toned voice.
   b. Use visual means of communication, such as gestures, cards, word lists.
   c. If the person has a hearing aid, clean the ear mold daily with soap and water, and check the cannula daily for patency.
   d. Replace old batteries before the expiration date, record the installation of new hearing aid batteries.
   e. Arrange for audiometric testing if necessary.

LEARNING CHECK

1. Glaucoma is characterized by a gradual loss of _____ _____ .
2. If untreated, glaucoma will result in _____ .
3. A person with cataracts often experiences a marked increase in the ability to _____ ; but this is transient.
4. All hearing losses should be evaluated by _____ _____ .
5. _____ is a common hearing disorder among older persons.

10

Metabolic Disorders

Common health problems affecting the endocrine system may occur from a disturbance in the secretion of hormones. A deficiency in a specific hormone usually results from destruction of the gland, cancer, infection, or from inadequate stimulation. An excess in a specific hormone usually results from tumors, hyperplasia, or hypertrophy. The purpose of this chapter is to provide the nurse with potential nursing diagnoses and appropriate nursing interventions for clients experiencing health problems of the endocrine system.

DIABETES MELLITUS

The peak age incidence of newly diagnosed diabetes is 60 to 70. Classic symptoms, such as thirst, sweating, polyuria, and tachycardia, are often absent among older persons. Behavior disorders, confusion, nocturnal headache, and slurred speech are usually the first symptoms. Decreased vision, intermittent claudication, numbing of the extremities, and shiny hairless skin over the lower legs may also be indicative of diabetes mellitus. The renal threshold for glucose increases with age; older persons can be hyperglycemic without "spilling" sugar in the urine according to Sundwall, Rolando, and Thorne (1981, p. 142).

Diabetes mellitus is classified into two types: Type I, insulin-dependent diabetes mellitus (IDDM); and Type II, non-insulin-dependent diabetes mellitus (NIDDM). Older persons generally develop NIDDM because the body cells are not receptive or sensitive to the insulin produced by the body, even though adequate insulin may be produced.

Hypoglycemia is usually a greater threat to older diabetics than hyperglycemia. Additionally, older diabetics tend to develop hyperglycemic hyperosmotic nonketonic coma (HHNK) rather than ketoacidosis when the diabetes is out of control.

The primary focus of medical management is on dietary management and medication administration. Recognition of the person's individual signs and symptoms of hypoglycemia and hyperglycemia is most important in order to control the diabetic process.

Potential Nursing Diagnoses

1. Potential for fluid volume deficit due to hyperosmolarity
2. Alteration in nutrition, less than body requirements, related to inadequate glucose reaching the cells
3. Potential for impairment of skin integrity due to compromised circulation

Potential Nursing Interventions

1. Maintain adequate hydration:
   a. Assess skin for decreased turgor, observe mucous membranes for dryness.
   b. Offer and provide fluids frequently.
2. Maintain adequate glucose levels:
   a. Administer hypoglycemic agent at the same time every day.
   b. If insulin mixtures are used, prepare the injection immediately before administration, unless a special stabilized premixed insulin product is prescribed.
   c. Rotate and record insulin injection sites.
   d. Do not rely on urine dipstick or tape tests as indicators

of hyperglycemia, since the renal threshold for glucose may be altered or elevated.

3. Maintain skin integrity:
    a. Apply lanolin-based lotion or oil daily to the skin; avoid overdrying the skin by too much bathing.
    b. Provide daily foot care. The feet need to be soaked in tepid water and gently massaged. The nails are cut straight across.
    c. Arrange for podiatric care if necessary.

HYPOTHYROIDISM

Hypothyroidism is a common health problem of older persons, and its development may be overlooked because the symptoms are not specific. Weakness, cold intolerance, memory impairment, weight gain, facial edema, hair loss, dry skin, chest pain, and constipation are among the symptoms frequently reported. Myxedema coma, or profound hypothyroidism, is a medical emergency requiring admission to an acute care facility. Myxedema often follows a serious illness, such as myocardial infarction, gastrointestinal bleeding, stroke, or infection. Hypothermia is a chief symptom of myxedema (Sundwall et al., 1981, p. 139–140).

Medical diagnosis of hypothyroidism is made through laboratory testing, and medical treatment is thyroid replacement therapy.

Potential Nursing Diagnoses

1. Alteration in cardiac output due to decreased heart rate
2. Alteration in sensory perception, related to coldness

Potential Nursing Interventions

1. Monitor closely for vascular collapse:
    a. Monitor heart rate, rhythm, blood pressure.

    b. Auscultate heart, chest sounds for development of pericardial, pleural effusions.

2. Keep the person warm, avoid chilling:
    a. Monitor temperature.
    b. Avoid the use of heating pads, electric blankets, which may warm too rapidly.
    c. Provide extra clothing, blankets; encourage wearing knit leg warmers.

HYPERTHYROIDISM

Hyperthyroidism is less common than hypothyroidism among older persons, but it is a health problem that also may be overlooked. Persons who have hyperthyroidism often complain of fatigue, leg cramps, palpitations, nervousness, and heat intolerance. Weight loss, exophthalmos (protrusion of the eyes), elevated temperature, and cardiac arrythmias are often noted. Schteingart (1978, p. 699) emphasizes that clinical manifestations of hyperthyroidism may be less obvious in elderly patients in whom it may present as an arrhythmia and heart failure. Medical diagnosis is made by laboratory testing, and medical treatment is directed at suppressing thyroid function.

Potential Nursing Diagnosis

1. Alteration in nutrition, less than body requirements, due to increased metabolism
2. Potential for eye injury due to protrusion of the eyes
3. Alteration in cardiac output due to increased rate

Potential Nursing Interventions

1. Maintain adequate nutrition, body weight:
    a. Increase number of meals and snacks.
    b. Weigh at least once a week and document.

2. Protect eyes from corneal damage, injury:
   a. Encourage use of dark glasses if person is exposed to bright light or sunlight.
   b. If eyelids do not close completely, apply protective eye patch during the night.
   c. Instill drops as ordered.
3. Monitor for increased cardiac workload:
   a. Assess vital signs, including temperature.
   b. Keep room cool.
   c. Apply cool compresses to forehead if person complains of excessive heat.
   d. Do not give aspirin to reduce fever; aspirin increases thyroxine levels (Doenges, Jeffries, & Moorhouse, 1984, p. 469).

LEARNING CHECK

1. Hypoglycemia is a greater threat to older diabetics than _____ .
2. Older diabetics are more apt to develop HHNK than _____ .
3. The renal threshold for glucose _____ with age.
4. Persons with hypothyroidism often complain of being _____ .
5. _____ _____ , profound hypothyroidism, is a grave medical emergency.
6. Signs of hyperthyroidism may present as an _____ and _____ _____ in the older adult.

11

Skin Disorders

The major function of the skin is protective. Other functions include heat regulation, sensation, and body image. Gradual changes occur in the skin of the older person, especially skin surfaces exposed to solar and environmental traumas. A common health problem involving the integumentary system of the older person is often the development of decubiti. The purpose of this chapter is to guide the nurse to possible nursing interventions for clients with the nursing diagnoses of alteration in skin integrity, actual or potential.

DECUBITUS ULCERS

The immobile aged are high-risk candidates for the development of decubiti due to fragility of the skin, decreased blood supply, reduced pressure sensation, and poor nutrition. Decubitus ulcers are best treated by prevention and through maintenance of skin care protocols.

Identification of those persons who are apt to develop decubiti is the first step in prevention. Special mattresses, such as egg crate types, or special pads can be used to avoid or reduce pressure. The skin must be kept scrupulously clean and dry. Care must be taken, however, not to overdry the skin. Soap with high fat content should be used. The skin must be kept well lubricated.

Immobile or bedfast persons must be turned and repositioned frequently to prevent pressure. Persons in wheelchairs or gerichairs should be repositioned more frequently than bedfast persons due to unequal distribution of body weight. An individual, written turning schedule or checklist should be used to ensure repositioning. All bony prominences should be gently massaged at the turning times.

Vigorous work is necessary to achieve healing once the skin is broken or an ulcer is formed. Assessment of the broken area or ulcer is the first step in the healing protocol. Byrne and Feld (1984) suggest classifying decubiti into four stages. In Stage I the epidermis and dermis are damaged, but not destroyed. In Stage II the epidermis and dermis are destroyed and damage has reached the subcutaneous layer. In Stage III the subcutaneous layer is destroyed, and there is cavity formation. In Stage IV muscle and bone tissue are involved, and skin tissues and structures are decayed.

Written records and diagrams or photographs of any decubiti must be kept. Culture and sensitivity studies of broken areas also are necessary.

A variety of decubitus ulcer treatments are available. Some of the treatment modalities include the application of antacid preparations or sugar; the application of karaya materials; the application of wet-to-dry dressings; the application of semipermeable membranes; and the application of enzymatic debriding substances. Enzymatic debriding agents should not be used unless necrotic tissue is present. Arnell (1983) recommends that hydrogen peroxide should be used to cleanse ulcers when a debriding agent is used; however, acetic acid ($1/2\%$ to 1%) should be used for cleansing if the ulcer is infected with a *Pseudomonas* species. After cleansing, the affected area must be well rinsed with normal saline.

The important issue in the nursing management of decubiti is that the selected treatment be done consistently and effectively and that the selected treatment be periodically evaluated.

STASIS ULCERS

Although the development of stasis ulcers in the lower extremities is due to chronic arterial or chronic venous insufficiency (peripheral vascular disease), it is discussed in this section rather than with the cardiovascular diseases because the chief nursing problem is that of impaired skin integrity. Like decubitus ulcers, these ulcers are easier to prevent than heal, and they require intensive nursing management.

Stasis ulcers are the result of chronic impairment of blood flow to or from the feet. According to Bates (1983, p. 318–319), the ulcer is usually located on the inner aspect of the ankle when the impairment is due to chronic venous insufficiency. The surrounding skin has a brownish discoloration. This condition is known as stasis dermatitis. The foot becomes cyanotic when it is lowered. The pain is not usually severe.

When the ulcer is due to chronic arterial insufficiency, it is usually seen on the lateral areas of the ankle or shin; the toes and feet may also be involved. Pain is usually severe. The surrounding skin is pale and shiny. Redness results when the foot is lowered.

The first step in the nursing management of stasis ulcers is assessment. Written records, diagrams, or photographs of the wounds are maintained. Pulses and the color of the extremity are also recorded. The affected extremity must be protected from injury. Bed cradles and special pads should be used to avoid pressure and shearing by bed linens. A culture and sensitivity should be obtained. Aseptic technique must be used when dressings are changed.

Enzymatic ointment may be prescribed to remove necrotic tissue. See the recommendations for cleansing agents listed in the "Decubitus Ulcer" section of this chapter.

Compression bandages (gelatin compression boot, Unna's boot) are sometimes prescribed for the management of venous stasis ulcers. Solid (1984) cautions that these treatments should not be used if the ulcer is arterial or if there is weeping eczema or cellulitis. The boot is applied following the manufacturer's direction. Circulation is observed frequently after application. The lesion may be covered every 3 to 4 days initially, with longer intervals between changes as healing takes place.

LEARNING CHECK

1. Decubitus ulcers may be classified into _____ stages.
2. Stasis ulcers that occur on the inner aspect of the ankle are usually due to _____ insufficiency.
3. Stasis ulcers that occur on the lateral areas of the lower extremities are usually due to _____ insufficiency.
4. Pain is usually severe when the ulcer is due to chronic _____ insufficiency.
5. Brownish discoloration on the lower part of the leg is called _____ _____ .

Part II References

Armstrong, M., & Cleary, M. (1982). Physiology of aging: Part II. In *Advances in geriatric long-term care nursing*. (Available from One Aldwyn Center, CN Box 7, Villanova, PA.)

Arnell, I. (1983). Treating decubitus ulcers. *Nursing 83, 13*(6), 55–56.

Autry, D., Lauzon, F., & Holliday, P. (1984). The voiding record: An aid in decreasing incontinence. *Geriatric Nursing, 5*(1), 22–25.

Bates, B. (1983). *A guide to physical examination* (3rd ed.). New York: McGraw-Hill.

Billings, D., & Stokes, L. (1982). *Medical surgical nursing*. St Louis: Mosby.

Blake, D. (1981). Physical assessment of the aged: Differentiating normal and abnormal change. In I.M. Burnside (Ed.), *Nursing and the aged* (2nd ed.). New York: McGraw-Hill.

Byrne, N., & Feld, M. (1984). Preventing and treating decubitus ulcers. *Nursing 84, 14*(4), 55–56.

Carotenuto, R., & Bullock, J. (1980). *Physical assessment of the gerontologic client*. Philadelphia: Davis.

Carroll, M. (1984). Infection control in long term care. *Geriatric Nursing, 5*(2), 100–103.

Davis, M., Eshleman, D., & McKay, M. (1982). *The relaxation and stress reduction workbook*. Oakland, CA: New Harbinger Publications.

Doenges, M., Jeffries, W., & Moorhouse, F. (1984). *Nursing care plans: Nursing diagnoses in planning patient care*. Philadelphia: Davis.

Eliopoulos, C. (1979). *Gerontological nursing*. New York: Harper and Row.

Ettinger, R. (1982, April). *Dental care and the elderly*. Eighth Annual Gerontology Institute, Springfield, IL.

Farber, S. (1982). *Neurorehabilitation: A multisensory approach*. Philadelphia: Saunders.

Howser, D. (1976). Ice water for MI patients! Why not? *American Journal of Nursing, 76*(3), 432–434.

Jacobs, R. (1981). Physical changes in the aged. In M. O'Hara-Devereaux, L. Andrus, & C. Scott (Eds.), *Eldercare* (pp. 31–47). New York: Grune and Stratton.

Keene, J. & Anderson, C. (1982). Hip fractures in the elderly. *Journal of the American Medical Association, 248*(5), 564–567.

Kintzel, K. (1977). *Advanced concepts in clinical nursing* (2nd ed.). Philadelphia: Lippincott.

Mace, N. & Rabins, P. (1981). *The thirty-six-hour day*. Baltimore: Johns Hopkins Press.

Mager-O'Conner, E. (1984). How to identify and remove fecal impactions. *Geriatric Nursing, 5*(3), 158–161.

Moehrlin, B., Wolanin, M., & Burnside, I. (1981). Nutrition and the elderly. In I.M. Burnside (Ed.), *Nursing and the aged* (2nd ed.) (pp. 323–348). New York: McGraw-Hill.

Morgan, W., Thomas, C., & Schuster, M. (1981). Gastrointestinal system. In M.O. O'Hara-Devereaux, L. Andrus, & C. Scott (Eds.), *Eldercare* (pp. 199–215). New York: Grune and Stratton.

Podlone, M., & Millikan, C. (1981). Neurology. In M. O'Hara-Devereaux, L. Andrus, & C. Scott (Eds.), *Eldercare* (pp. 115–134). New York: Grune and Stratton.

Prillaman, P., & Junk, R. (1984). *Alzheimer's disease: What you need to know.* Available from the Central Illinois Chapter of the ADRDA, 807 N. Main St., Bloomington, IL 61701.

Richards, M. (1982). Osteoporosis. *Geriatric Nursing, 3*(2), 98–102.

Rosal-Greif, V. (1982). Drug-induced dyskinesias. *American Journal of Nursing, 82*(1), 66–69.

Rosenzweig, M. R., & Leiman, A. L. (1982). *Physiological psychology* (pp. 652–653). Lexington, MA: D.C. Heath.

Rossman, I. (1981). Human aging changes. In I.M. Burnside (Ed.), *Nursing and the aged* (2nd ed.) (pp. 30–40). New York: McGraw-Hill.

Sahs, A., Hartman, E., & Aronson, S. (1976). *Guidelines for stroke care* (DHEW Publication No. HRA 76–14017). Washington, DC: U.S. Government Printing Office.

Schteingart, D. (1978). Endocrinology and metabolism: Principles of pathophysiology. In S. Price and L. Wilson (Eds.), *Pathophysiology: Clinical concepts of disease processes* (pp. 648–696). New York: McGraw-Hill.

Shannon, M. (1984). Five famous fallacies about pressure sores. *Nursing 84, 14*(10), 34–41.

Solid, R. (1984). Give venous leg ulcers the boot. *Nursing 84, 14*(11), 52–53.

Sundwall, D., Rolando, J., & Thorn, G. (1981). Endocrine and metabolic. In M. O'Hara-Devereaux, L. Andrus, & C. Scott (Eds.), *Eldercare* (pp. 135–147). New York: Grune and Stratton.

Taisch, E., Taisch, D., & Metz, H. (1981). Problems of the eyes. In M. O'Hara-Devereaux, L. Andrus, & C. Scott (Eds.), *Eldercare* (pp. 259–275). New York: Grune and Stratton.

U. S. Department of Commerce, Bureau of the Census. (1975). *Statistical Abstract of the United States 1975* (No. 86, 1975). Washington, DC: U. S. Government Printing Office.

Walraven, B., Malik, P., & Cyr, D. (1981). Hematology. In M. O'Hara-Devereaux, L. Andrus, & C. Scott (Eds.), *Eldercare* (pp. 235–246). New York: Grune and Stratton.

Williams, H., McDonald, E., Daggett, M., Schut, B., & Buckwalter, K. (1983). Treating dysphagia. *Journal of Gerontological Nursing, 9*(12), 638–647.

Wolanin, M., & Phillips, L. (1981). *Confusion: Prevention and care.* St. Louis: Mosby.

PART III

Focusing on the Whole Person

The purposes of this part are to:
1. Discuss developmental tasks associated with aging
2. Discuss psychosocial health problems commonly experienced by older persons
3. Suggest nursing diagnoses applicable to actual or potential psychosocial health problems
4. Cite components of adequate nutrition among older persons
5. Discuss measures nurses may utilize to promote sound nutrition among elders
6. Discuss certain features of a facilitative environment for institutionalized elders
7. Cite measures nurses can employ to foster a facilitative environment in the home

12

Psychosocial Aspects of Elders' Care

Jerry D. Durham, R.N., Ph.D.

Elders comprise the largest group of persons for whom nurses provide care in hospitals, nursing homes, home health, and in the general community. As the American population ages, health resources will be increasingly directed toward meeting the needs of this growing population. In 1900, 1 of every 25 Americans was 65 or older; in 1980 every 9th American (or 25 million persons) had reached this age. By the year 2000, 35 million persons will have reached this age, and by 2025 the number will have grown to over 58 million (Brody, 1985).

A variety of changes and developmental stressors among elders predispose them to mental distress or illness. It was estimated in 1980 that approximately 30% of Americans over age 65 needed some mental health intervention and that more than half of the frail elderly residing in long-term care facilities had diagnosable psychiatric disorders (Kermis, 1986). Risk of mental dysfunction or illness increases significantly after age 75. Brody (1985), referring to 1980 statistics from the Center on Aging of the National Institute of Mental Health, reports that mental illness is more prevalent among elders than young adults; psychosis increases significantly after age 65 and again after age 75; dementia is believed to be the fourth leading cause of death; suicide is prominent among elders; and significant chronic ailments among elders contribute to negative psychological reactions. She points out that reduced opportunities for social interaction, reduced income and poverty, role losses, and multiple personal losses contribute significantly to mental health problems in elders. There is presently both an undersupply of personnel to meet these needs and a lack of emphasis upon these health needs within this population.

In spite of these significant problems, elders often experience emotional difficulties for long periods before receiving treatment. According to Waxman and Carner (1984), utilization studies show that while persons over 65 comprise 11% of the population, they constitute only 4% to 5% of admissions to psychiatric emergency departments. Studies of inpatient psychiatric facilities and outpatient psychiatric services reveal a similar pattern of underutilization of mental health services by elders. These findings would seem to suggest that nurses may play significant roles in identifying elders with mental health difficulties and in providing effective treatment.

Brody (1985) has identified barriers to mental health care of elders to include reimbursement structures under federal programs and other financial barriers; fragmented, disorganized health and social services for elders; inadequately trained mental health professionals interested in problems related to aging; negative attitudes toward the aging; transportation and other problems of accessibility; and "turf-guarding" by agencies working to protect reduced resources. Elders may not seek treatment because they lack awarenesss of mental health services; they fear they will be stigmatized; they have low self-esteem, which deters them from seeking help; and they believe that their suffering is a normal part of aging.

For several reasons nurses are in a position to greatly enhance the psychosocial health of elders. Nurses have greater contact with elders than any other group of licensed health professionals. Recent surveys strongly suggest that elders, like Americans from other age groups, trust nurses. Nurses come from an educational background that prepares them to use excellent communication skills in establishing and maintaining a trusting relationship; furthermore, increasing numbers of nurses have advanced knowledge of issues and concerns affecting elders. Finally, nurses have demonstrated a willingness to accept the roles of advocate and change agent for elders.

Considering the growing number of elders in the United States, nurses need to understand elders' psychosocial health as influenced by various factors, such as the physical aging process, illness, developmental changes, and the availability of support systems. Moreover, nurses need to adopt a holistic view of elders in order to fully assist them in meeting their health care needs; those accepting this view readily see the close relationship betweeen mental and physical health. According to Karpowich (1980), nurses working with elders have the following role responsibilities:

1. Strengthening elders' abilities to maintain and promote their own health.
2. Supervising and coordinating care of common health problems and chronic illnesses.
3. Evaluating and planning the treatment of illness.
4. Referring for specialized health care when appropriate.
5. Collaborating with other health care agencies.

Psychotherapy with elders having a diagnosed psychiatric disorder is best provided by health professionals with special training in these skills. Increasing numbers of nurses with such skills now work in the role of private practitioner or clinical nurse specialist. Many work therapeutically with elders with specific mental health disorders (Edinberg, 1985; Horton, 1982). However, most elders cared for by nurses do not require psychotherapy; rather, they need skillful nursing care based upon knowledge, insight, and a sincere and caring attitude. Care of elders should include observations that identify deviations from normalcy, with care being primarily directed toward the prevention of health problems, including those of a psychosocial nature.

Kermis (1986) has noted the core knowledge and competencies for individuals trained to deal with the mental health needs of older persons. These recommendations, based upon the work of Eisdorfer and Cohen (1982) and Smyer and Gatz (1979), deserve the attention of nurses working with elders:

1. An understanding of normal aging processes, including knowledge of the myths and realities of personality and adjustment processes in late life, including:
   a. Normative crises of late life
   b. Personality patterns
   c. Intellectual skills
   d. Myths and stereotypes of old age
2. An understanding of the ways in which older persons cope with stress, including the causes and mechanisms of stress, as well as defenses used to deal with psychological trauma.
3. An understanding of the pathology encountered in old age, including knowledge of psychological disorders that are more prevalent in old age. Issues to be dealt with include:
   a. Symptoms of these disorders
   b. Suspected etiologies
   c. Appropriate treatments for disorders
   d. Differentiation of depression and dementia

4. An understanding of basic communication skills to use with older people in mental distress.
5. An understanding of methods useful in dealing with other human service professionals and family members on behalf of elderly clients.

Many gerontological nurses already possess this knowledge base and these competencies. Others, depending upon their professional roles, may wish to develop these through the educational approaches noted earlier.

THEORIES AND CONCEPTS RELEVANT TO ELDERS' MENTAL HEALTH

An overview of some of the relevant theories related to psychosocial health can help gerontological nurses in their work with elders. Karpowich (1980) has listed 23 universal needs of elders that take into account their needs for independence, a sense of purpose, self-confidence, and self-esteem. These needs include a meaningful and puposeful life, companionship and recreation, privacy, control over life situations, life and death with dignity, meaningful relationships, sexual expression, and maintenance of peer and family roles. To assist them in meeting these needs, elders want to be cared for by nurses who are kind and caring (e.g., friendly attitude, good manners, and a mutual trusting friendship); who listen well and say the right thing in the right way; who respect their dignity, right to privacy, and desire for self-determination; and who maintain a professional presence (Grau, 1984).

The existence of universal needs among elders recognizes that they, like the more youthful in American society, have not merely entered the last developmental stage of life in which they passively await death. A more dynamic view of the developmental processes inherent in aging assists nurses who work with elders. Gress and Bahr (1984) maintain that elders "should not be deprived of the opportunity to continue their pursuit of personhood simply because of their age" (p. 38). In their overview of various developmental perspectives, these authors cite five types of aging:

1. Biological aging, which involves changes in structure and function of the body over the life span.
2. Psychological aging, which involves behavioral changes, changes in self-perception, and reaction to biological changes.
3. Functional aging, which measures capacities of individuals for functioning in society as compared with others of the same age.
4. Sociological aging, which involves roles and habits of society.
5. Spiritual aging, which concerns changes of self and perceptions of self, of the relationship of self to others, of the place of the self in the world, and of the self's world view.

Each type of aging, presumably experienced by all persons, is subject to change and to shifts in priority at various times throughout life.

According to Havighurst's developmental task theory (1953), the tasks of later maturity are to adjust to decreasing physical strength and health; adjust to retirement and reduced income; adjust to death of a spouse; establish an affiliation with one's age group; adopt and adapt social roles in a flexible way; and establish satisfactory living arrangements. By understanding these developmental tasks and evaluating elders' abilities to meet these tasks, the nurse can identify actual and potential psychosocial/developmental difficulties and use available resources to resolve them.

To help elders achieve their highest level of mental health, the nurse might also consider implementing the five steps of

Kuypers and Bengtson's (1973) "Social Reconstruction Syndrome," which seeks to prevent the loss of identity and independence which can accompany aging:

1. Reducing susceptibility and promoting self-confidence.
2. Reducing dependence and increasing self-reliance.
3. Self-labeling as being capable or able.
4. Building and maintaining coping skills.
5. Internalizing a view of oneself as an effective human being.

Stereotyping older persons is a serious problem that, unfortunately, occurs among some nurses. According to Vander Zyl (1983), elders become more unique as they age; yet their unique needs may go unmet. They often are treated not as unique individuals, but rather as if there were a single, typical older person. Nurses, as members of society at large, may unintentionally propagate long-held myths about elders: They are an unproductive, senile, sexless, rigid, emotionally fragile, incompetent, and homogenous lot. A number of studies (Buschman, Burns, & Jones, 1981; Heller & Walsch, 1976; Smith, Jepson, & Perloff, 1982; Wilhite & Johnson, 1976) have focused upon stereotypes that often negatively influence care of elders. According to Dolinsky (1984), such views can lead some caregivers to treat elders as infants, rather than as mature adults, thereby encouraging them to become less competent and self-sufficient than they might otherwise be. Elders who accept these views and resulting treatment eventually act accordingly. Their behaviors, and those of their caregivers, are reinforced by stereotyped attitudes, normal dependencies of aging, institutional characteristics, and individual client characteristics.

In addition to stereotyped views of elders that impinge upon their care, some caregivers consider aging a stigma, reflecting an attitude that is too frequently supported by

American society's emphasis upon beauty and youth. Anything that elicits a negative attitude can be said to carry a stigma (e.g., antisocial acts, mental illness, and physical unattractiveness). Stigmatization of elders can lead to distancing behaviors by caregivers, which furthers elders' isolation.

Johnson and Grant (1985) underscore how the nursing home environment can negatively affect mental health of residents, depending upon such factors as the privacy provided, the rigidity of scheduling and controls, access to personal property, and the extent of isolation from the outside world. They have catalogued the following effects:

1. Deindividuation (reduced capacity for thought, action, and self-direction).
2. Disculturation (loss of lifelong rules and behaviors that provide the individual with sources of self-affirmation).
3. Emotional, social, and physical damage.
4. Estrangement (isolation from the outside world).
5. Isolation from society in general.
6. Stimulus deprivation (deadening of the senses of an individual who has grown accustomed to the institutional environment).

They suggest that these effects may be caused by nursing home resident selection biases, preadmission effects, institutional environmental effects, and changes in the environment following relocation. Gubrium (1975), Krause (1982), Laird (1979), and Moss and Halamandaris (1977) have also contributed interesting analyses of the impact of nursing homes upon residents.

The negative impact of nursing homes upon elders would seem to reinforce "disengagement" of elders as described by Cumming and Henry (1961). According to this theory, aging persons gradually and inevitably withdraw (or disengage) from society, thereby minimizing social disruption when death occurs. Rose (1968) believes that a number of forces operating in society today counteract disengagement of the elderly. These have been summarized to include large numbers of healthy and vigorous persons over 65 years of age; elders' increased economic security, which promotes leisure activities; active involvement of elders in activities that promote their status and privileges; earlier retirement, which allows elders to develop activities and relationships that extend further into late life; and increased "engagement" opportunities for elders.

It is not possible to postulate principles that guide the nursing care of all elders under all circumstances since they, like persons from other age groups, have a great variety of characteristics and needs. However, Gress and Bahr (1984) have summarized beliefs that can guide nurses in their contact with elders regardless of the setting. These beliefs, if endorsed and considered in the nursing process, can have a profoundly positive effect upon the nurse-client relationship and upon the mental health of elders. Briefly stated, these authors believe that elders:

1. Are worthy of respect and entitled to dignity.
2. Are beings created by an external force.
3. Experience life, death, and a wide range of human emotions.
4. Represent an integrated, organized whole; interact with their environment.
5. Are subject to changes of aging which may diminish their function but not their value.
6. Are in a state of change.
7. Are interested in learning health-related information to maintain and promote their wellness.

By recognizing and adopting these beliefs, nurses can form attitudes and values that promote a view of elders as worthwhile, unique persons and can drive back myths about aging that have for too long perpetuated unhealthy adaptation in American society.

ASSESSING ELDERS' PSYCHOSOCIAL STATUS

Assessment represents the first step in the nursing process and forms the basis for subsequent diagnosis, planning, implementation of nursing actions, and evaluation of those actions. Assessment, according to Edinberg (1985), allows the examiner to decrease the amount of extraneous information about a client's functioning, to decrease incorrect judgments about a client's status and functioning, and to provide a common framework and language for sharing findings. Kane and Kane (1981) have summarized the purposes of systematic assessment of elders:

1. To document the individual's problems.
2. To pinpoint conditions needing additional services/support.
3. To document changes in functioning; to accurately diagnose/document problems.
4. To provide a basis for monitoring progress.
5. To assist in predicting outcomes or decisions in case management.
6. To obtain information in an efficient manner.

A number of instruments and approaches can assist the nurse in assessing elders' psychosocial status, functional abilities, sources of support, and behavior. Such data are valuable in assisting the nurse to construct interventions that hold the potential to significantly improve the lives of elders whom the nurse treats.

At least 20 tests exist for measuring mental status alone.

More than one approach may be appropriate, depending upon the setting, the examiner's skill, time limitations, client cooperation, and the purpose of the examination. Mental status assessment is particularly important in long-term work with clients in nursing homes and in community settings. Most mental status examinations explore the individual's cognitive functioning, including orientation, recent and distant memory, perceptual ability, psychomotor ability, attention span/concentration, problem solving/judgment, social intactness, reaction time, learning ability, and intelligence. Common instruments used for assessing cognitive functioning include the Mental Status Questionnaire (MSQ) (Kermis, 1986; Wolanin & Phillips, 1981) and the Short Portable Mental Status Questionnaire (SPMSQ) (Pfeiffer, 1975).

A number of authors have also endorsed the use of the Bender's Face-Hand Test of Orientation (FHT) to augment the MSQ and the SPMSQ (1981, p. 190). With the FHT, the client is simultaneously stimulated on the hand and cheek in at least 10 trials. Errors in these trials are generally indicative of brain damage. These three tests are equally administered and have proven particularly effective in screening out individuals with organic brain syndromes. Because some estimates indicate that as many as 50 to 70% of elders in institutions suffer from some form of cognitive or affective impairment and because common reasons for the admission of elders to nursing homes include "senility" or organic brain syndromes (Lincoln, 1984), means to identify such difficulties are of importance. Causes of confused states are discussed elsewhere in this book and by Palmateer and McCartney (1985), Wolanin and Phillips (1981), and Wolanin (1983). Measurement of social functioning, according to Johnson and Grant (1985), is concerned with the extent to which an older person has the resources to avoid institutionalization; the level of social competence necessary to maintain social interaction; or, within institutional settings, the evaluation of the degree of social interaction. The following indices of social functioning are items frequently assessed: demographic characteristics, social contacts, health status self-rating, living arrangements, social participation, satisfaction with social supports, economic status, and self-maintenance of daily living with social supports.

Still another useful approach is identified by Morgan and Morgan (1980). Besides the standard mental health status examination, the authors suggest questioning clients about life stressors. Because many elders have experienced major developmental and life-event stressors, nurses should consider assessing these factors. Common stressors that the authors describe in detail include the following: personal injury or illness, marital stressors, stresses of parenting, stressors of employment, financial stressors, environmental stressors, other interpersonal stressors, and other life stressors.

Assessment of affective functioning is directed toward uncovering depression, suicidal risk, and demoralization. As many as 15 to 20% of the elderly population are estimated to experience depression serious enough to warrant treatment, according to Shamoian (1985). Depression in elders may be manifested in a variety of ways, which can mimic or be misdiagnosed as a physical illness; moreover, physical illness can contribute to or exacerbate depression. Many depressed elders present with cognitive dysfunctions that are mistaken for dementia; unfortunately, no clear methods exist to distinguish pseudomentia in the form of depression from dementia.

Although the elderly account for only 12% of the population, they constitute 25% of the successful suicides in this country. Suicide rates among older women are among the highest of any age group, while the rate for men increases with age (Kermis, 1986). In comparison to elders who live independently, fewer nursing home residents commit suicide because many are physically unable or lack the means to do so. Because their appeals for psychological help are frequently inhibited or masked and because many care providers do not recognize indicators of suicide risk, many elders' first suicide attempts are frequently successful (Kermis, 1986). Those elders at highest risk of committing suicide include those recently widowed; those living alone; those with a chronic debilitating illness; and those with a history of drug abuse and suicide attempts (Shamoian, 1985). A screening test, the Geriatric Depression Scale, developed by Brink, Yesavage, Lum, Heersma, Adey, and Rose (1982), is a short, easily administered test that may be useful in a variety of clinical settings.

AN OVERVIEW OF ELDERS' PSYCHOSOCIAL HEALTH

In addition to the physical and cognitive changes with which many elders must cope, multiple physical, mental, social, and economic losses may also inflict emotional fear, grief or depression, anger, dependency, helplessness, sense of failure, humiliation, and shame. These losses, both anticipated and unplanned, are often multiple: the loss of vigor and health; the loss of functional abilities or senses; the loss of the spouse, children, friends, or pets; the loss of significant social bonds; the loss of employment because of retirement or illness; the loss of income; the loss of family roles; the loss of home; and loss of attractiveness, sexuality, or sexual expression. This sense of loss may be more greatly felt by elders forced to enter nursing homes because of declining health. Depending upon the individual's previous coping abilities, sources of support, and general state of health, these losses may exact an onerous toll on a person's mental health. The losses may result in grief, depression, anxiety, stress reactions, withdrawal, and a diminished desire to continue living.

Among the estimated 1.2 million elders living in institutions, both physical and mental illnesses are prominent. Rovner and Rabins (1985) point out that over the past 20 years the number of nursing home residents has quadrupled. At the same time, the number of elders in long-term psychiatric hospitals has declined. These displaced individuals now occupy 8% of nursing home beds. According to Rovner and Rabins, mental disorders among nursing home residents are frequently misdiagnosed, undiagnosed, or diagnosed in a way that obscures treatable disorders. Dementia, discussed elsewhere within this text, is the most prevalent mental disorder among institutionalized older persons. The second most common mental disorder in nursing home residents is depression. A third, and often more disruptive problem among nursing home residents, is that of disordered behavior, manifested by irritability and explosiveness, wandering, sleeplessness, resisting nursing care and efforts to maintain hygiene, and yelling. Rovner and Rabins (1985) have suggested that at least part of these behavioral problems may stem from residents' impairments in their communication, their recognition of familiar faces and objects, and their performance of everyday activities.

To improve the mental health of residents of nursing homes whose caregivers are largely nonprofessional, Rovner and Rabins (1985) suggest a multifaceted approach that includes increased psychiatric consultation; improved use of nonphysician mental health specialists; the establishment of accurate psychiatric diagnoses; in-service education focused on psychiatric disorders; emotional support for families of residents; encouragement of family participation in daily care; and increased activity therapy to improve mood, increase socialization, prevent physical deterioration, and provide stimulation.

Feldman (1982) and Madalon, Weiner, and Amenta (1984) have provided insight into the stress that can result from elders' sudden relocation, including hospital admission. Unplanned hospital admission can also lead to a state of crisis in elders as a result of their distorted perception of the event, inadequate support from significant others and the environment, and inadequate coping mechanisms. The resulting effects are often increased anxiety and depression, helplessness and disorganization, and rapid mental deterioration. Elders whose mental health status was compromised prior to hospital admission may become severly confused, agitated, or psychotic. Other considerations that negatively affect the coping abilities and mental health of hospitalized elders include multisystem disease, poor nutritional status, diminished overall strength, deleterious drug interactions, lengthy hospital stays, and "ageism" (i.e., prejudice against elders) (Ruskin, 1985). Common medical emergencies that precipitate elders' hospital admissions also contribute to their anxiety and to their mental deterioration. The combination of relocation stress, medical illness, and inadequate environmental support may require intervention by mental health specialists. Prevention of these reactions may often be accomplished by carefully assessing behavior, carefully monitoring vital signs and elimination, being knowledgeable of the effects of administered drugs, eliminating sensory deprivation/overload, and encouraging visits by significant others.

POTENTIAL NURSING DIAGNOSES

Several nursing diagnoses may describe potential or actual psychosocial problems related to aging. This list may include the following:

1. Anxiety
2. Impaired verbal communication
3. Ineffective individual coping
4. Diversional activity deficit
5. Fear

6. Alterations in family processes
7. Grieving
8. Powerlessness
9. Disturbance in self-concept
10. Sensory-perceptual impairment
11. Sleep pattern disturbance
12. Social isolation
13. Spiritual distress
14. Alterations in thought processes
15. Potential for violence

In addition to the above nursing diagnoses, numerous other diagnoses relevant to psychiatric illnesses are commonly used by mental health specialists, including nurses, as described in the American Psychiatric Association's *Diagnostic and Statistical Manual of Mental Disorders*, 3rd edition (1980).

COMMON PSYCHOSOCIAL STRESSORS AMONG ELDERS

The purpose of the following brief discussion is to alert nurses to psychosocial health problems commonly experienced by elders and to suggest approaches that may prevent or reduce the impact of these problems.

Relocation Stress

Relocation can cause rapid decline in elders. Elders are at high risk for residential, interinstitutional, and residential/institutional relocations. Involuntary moves in particular pose higher risks of unfavorable outcomes for elders, including an increased mortality rate. When an elder is transferred from nursing home to hospital, the results may include sensory alteration, immobility, social isolation, loss of control, and disorientation.

Relocation to a constraining environment (e.g., from a private residence to a nursing home) may result in feelings of helplessness, loss, and depression. Adjustment to relocation seems to be affected by the voluntary or involuntary nature of the move, the degree of environmental change, perception of the relocation, the amount and type of information provided about the relocation, the adequacy of coping mechanisms, and mental and physical health at the time of relocation.

Nurses can help elders adjust to relocation by beginning preparation for the move as soon as possible, by including elders as much as possible in the decisions about the move, by orienting them to the new environment and to persons within this setting prior to the relocation when possible, by providing information to elders and their families about the environment, by encouraging elders to take personal items to their new environment, by accompanying elders to the new environment, and by sharing pertinent information about elders with caregivers in the new environment.

Loss of Support Systems

There is evidence to suggest that elders' linkage to neighbors, kin, and friends can improve the quality of their lives; serve as a source of emotional support; help them to feel needed; assist them in coping with stressful life events; improve socialization, which lends continuity and structure to the life transtions; and link them to sources of formal services.

Support systems help individuals to socialize, carry out tasks of daily living, and provide assistance in times of illness and crisis. However, because many elders focus their mental activity inward, there is often a decrease in the scope of their social interactions, especially among those in institutional settings. Some experts believe that such changes associated with aging reflect elders' acceptance of termination of life. A number of factors may have reduced the informal support network of elders: loss of occupational role, which provided a network of acquaintances and friends; loss of mobility; loss of prestige and power; geographic distance from customary sources of support; and illness and death. Those who are very old often experience greater difficulty in maintaining a support system.

Residents of nursing homes may lack opportunities to establish meaningful bonds because many suffer communication impairments, cognitive deficits, or physical limitations. Other factors within nursing homes that discourage friendships include differences in ethnicity and social class among residents and caregivers, a physical layout that discourages movement, a fear that new friends will die, and an atmosphere that may stifle some residents' desire to form attachments.

Elders lacking social support systems are at risk for social isolation and enmeshment with caregivers. As a liaison between family and health care organizations, nurses can help to foster existing support systems and link elders to new ones to meet their health needs. Such linkage can improve elders' dignity and quality of life and maintain or re-establish family ties. Nurses can also direct their efforts toward the families of elders and offer suggestions and support them.

Death

Most older persons die in institutional settings where, unfortunately, caregivers are not always responsive to the needs of the dying or needs of their loved ones. Confronted by talk of death, professionals often provide false reassurance, deny that the person will die, change the topic, or intellectualize. Numerous fears are associated with death: pain, loss of control, changes in goals, fear of the death of others, fear of not being, fear of punishment in the afterlife, and impact upon survivors (Edinberg, 1985).

As elders recognize the finality of their lives, they need assistance in coping with the event. Edinberg (1985) suggests four principles to consider in working with the terminally ill:

1. Death is a phenomenon which is not and perhaps cannot be fully understood.
2. The goal of the work is adaptive rather than curative.
3. The client does the leading and the helper follows to assist the client to obtain what is needed.
4. The relationship is time-limited.

Edinberg also maintains that the major approach to work with the terminally ill is that of concern, care, and compassion. In assisting the dying client, the nurse first should be ready to listen to whatever the client, family, or significant other(s) have to say; second, the nurse should be knowledgeable about the diagnosis, prognosis, and care plan. The nurse should be prepared to recognize and handle reactions of denial and other forms of avoidance, anger, bargaining, depression, and acceptance, which may accompany the death process. Nurses who are themselves comfortable in discussing death can assist elders and their families to accept the inevitability of the situation and can promote a dignified death.

Since many nurses also work with elders who are bereaved or grieving, Edinberg's (1985) considerations for practitioners in their work with survivors are significant:

1. Attend to the bereaved before death.
2. Work with the survivors should commence within 3 days of the death.
3. Most survivors want to talk to a "listener."
4. Practitioners should explore negative feelings about the dead person.
5. The nurse is a sounding board who represents reality for the survivor.
6. Survivors' physical health and behavioral changes should receive attention.

Nurses should be aware that even normal grieving, often described as a process with multiple stages, may be a lengthy process, encompassing many months or even years. Common emotions and thoughts expressed by survivors include loneliness, numbness, being overwhelmed, sadness, anger, unreality, and a need for support (Whelan, 1985). Delayed, unresolved, or complicated grief can lead to alterations in survivors' mental and physical health and may require referral to a mental health specialist.

Diminished Self-Esteem

Hirst and Metcalf (1984) point out that without self-esteem, defined as a form of high evaluation of oneself based upon acceptance from others, one lacks courage to attempt new challenges and shrinks from interaction from others. High self-esteem in elders is demonstrated when they are able to integrate past with present and accept what is rather than what might have been. Hirst and Metcalf have listed the component parts of self-esteem to include roles, touch, meaningful relationships, sexuality, independence, and space. When these aspects of self-esteem are not acknowledged or met, elders may respond in several ways: by grieving over losses; by feeling useless; by feeling lonely; by feeling powerless, dependent, and disinterested; by withdrawing from others; and by resisting invasions into their territory as well as their personal and private spaces. While nursing home residents are at higher risk for diminished self-esteem than other elders, all older persons are probably at higher risk than those from other age groups.

Touch can promote the self-esteem of elders. While not every person is comfortable with touch, the literature suggests that touch is beneficial, conveys acceptance and caring, and fosters nurse-client rapport and client well-being (Seaman, 1982). Pets can also provide an alternate approach that encourages touching, reduces withdrawal, and helps to alleviate loneliness among persons living alone or within nursing homes (Erickson, 1985).

CONCLUSION

Nurses are in a unique position to assist elders in adapting to aging, to achieve, in the words of Gress and Bahr (1984), a "celebration of life." They can do this by helping elders to maintain their autonomy, to heighten their sense of self-esteem, to maintain support systems, to adapt to change, and to accept death. They can use their knowledge of elders' health needs and problems to identify potential or actual health problems and to design interventions that reduce the impact of these problems. They can help elders to adapt to a wide range of changes through various means: therapeutic listening, touch, reminiscing, reality orientation, and activity therapy. Finally, and perhaps most importantly, they can care for elders through the act of attending, that is, by sharing the gift of time and by using that time to instill in elders a sense of importance, worth, and value.

LEARNING CHECK

1. Nursing efforts to maintain and strengthen elders' ability to engage in self care will enhance their _____ , _____ .
2. _____ is a process that results in elders being treated as if there were a single, typical older person.
3. Reduced capacity for thought, action, and self-direction may be referred to as _____ .
4. A theory that holds that elders gradually and inevitably withdraw is known as _____ .

5. The two most significant mental impairments among elders are _____ and _____ .
6. Friends, families, and others are examples of elders' _____ _____ .
7. Roles, touch, sexuality, independence, and space are all component parts of _____ .

REFERENCES

American Psychiatric Association. (1980). *Diagnostic and statistical manual of mental disorders* (3rd ed.). Washington, DC: Author.

Bender, A. P. (1981). Face–hand test. In I. Burnside (Ed.), *Nursing and the aging* (p. 190). New York: McGraw-Hill.

Brink, T., Yesavage, J., Lum, O., Heersma, P., Adey, M., & Rose, T. (1982). Screening tests for geriatric depression. *Clinical Gerontologist, 1*, 37–43.

Brody, E. (1985). *Mental and physical health practices of older people*. New York: Springer.

Buschman, M., Burns, E., & Jones, F. (1981). Student nurses; attitudes toward the elderly. *Journal of Nursing Education, 20*, 7–10.

Cumming, E., & Henry, W. (1961). *Growing old*. Springfield, IL: Charles C Thomas.

Dolinsky, E. (1984). Infantilization of the elderly: An area of nursing research. *Journal of Gerontological Nursing, 10*(9), 12–19.

Edinberg, M. (1985). *Mental health practice with the elderly*. Englewood Cliffs, NJ: Prentice-Hall.

Eisdorfer, C., & Cohen, D. (1982). *Mental health care of the aging: A multidisciplinary curriculum for professional training*. New York: Springer.

Erickson, R. (1985). Companion animals and the elderly. *Geriatric Nursing, 6*(2), 92–96.

Feldman, A. (1982). Transfer: Nursing home to hospital. *Geriatric Nursing, 3*(5), 307–310.

Grau, L. (1984). What older adults expect from the nurse. *Geriatric Nursing, 5*(1), 14–18.

Gress, L., & Bahr, R. (1984). *The aging person: A holistic perspective*. St. Louis: Mosby.

Gubrium, J. (1975). *Living and dying at Murray Manor*. New York: St. Martin's Press.

Havighurst, R. (1953). *Human development and education*. New York: McKay.

Heller, B., & Walsch, F. (1976). Charming nursing students toward the aged: An experimental study. *Journal of Nursing Education, 15*(1), 9–17.

Hirst, S. & Metcalf, B. (1984). Promoting self-esteem. *Journal of Gerontological Nursing, 10*(2), 72–77.

Horton, A. (1982). *Mental health interventions for the aging.* New York: Praeger.

Johnson, C., & Grant, L. (1985). *The nursing home in American society.* Baltimore: Johns Hopkins.

Kane, R., & Kane, R. (1981). *Assessing the elderly: A practical guide to measurement.* Lexington, MA: Lexington Books.

Karpowich, D. (1980). Needs of elderly and health promotion. In M. Futrell, S. Brovender, E. McKinnon-Mullett, & H. Brower (Eds.), *Primary health care of the older adult* (pp. 25–48). North Scituate, MA: Duxbury.

Kermis, M. (1986). *Mental health in late life.* Boston: Jone & Bartlett.

Krause, D. (1982). *Home, bittersweet home.* Springfield, IL: Charles C Thomas.

Kuypers, J., & Bengston, V. (1973). Competence and social breakdown: A socio-psychological view of aging. *Human Development, 16,* 37–49.

Laird, C. (1979). *Limbo.* Novato, CA: Chandler and Sharp.

Lincoln, R. (1984). What do nurses know about confusion in the aged? *Journal of Gerontological Nursing, 10*(5), 26–32.

Madalon, A., Weiner, A., & Amenta, D. (1984). Successful relocation of elderly residents. *Geriatric Nursing, 5*(8), 356–360.

Morgan, A., & Morgan, M. (1980). *Manual of primary mental health care.* Philadelphia: Lippincott.

Moss, F., & Halamandaris, V. (1977). *Too old, too sick, too bad.* Germantown, MD: Aspen.

Palmateer, L., & McCartney, J. (1985). Do nurses know when patients have cognitive deficits? *Journal of Gerontological Nursing, 11*(2), 6–17.

Pfeiffer, E. (1975). A short portable mental status questionnaire for the assessment of organic brain deficit in elderly patients. *Journal of the American Geriatrics Society, 23,* 433–441.

Rose, A. (1968). A current theoretical issue. In B. Neugarten (Ed.), *Middle age and aging* (pp. 184–189). Chicago: University of Chicago Press.

Rovner, B., & Rabins, P. (1985). Mental illness among nursing home patients. *Hospital and Community Psychiatry, 36* (2), 119–128.

Ruskin, P. (1985). Geropsychiatric consultation in a university hospital: A report on 67 referrals. *American Journal of Psychiatry, 142*(3), 333–336.

Seaman, L. (1982). Affecting nursing touch. *Geriatric Nursing, 3*(3), 162–164.

Shamoian, C. (1985). Assessing depression in elderly patients. *Hospital and Community Psychiatry, 36*, 338–339.

Smith, S., Jepson, V., & Perloff, E. (1982). Attitudes of nursing care providers toward elderly patients. *Nursing and Health Care, 3*, 93–98.

Smyer, M., & Gatz, M. (1979). Aging and mental health: Business as usual? *American Psychologist, 34*, 240–246.

Vander Zyl, S. (1983). Psychotherapy with the elderly. *Journal of Psychosocial Nursing and Mental Health Services, 21*(10), 25–29.

Waxman, H., & Carner, E. (1984). Physicians' recognition, diagnosis, and treatment of mental disorders in elderly medical patients. *The Gerontologist, 24*, 593–597.

Whelan, E. (1985). Support for the survivor. *Geriatric Nursing, 6*(1), 21–23.

Wilhite, M., & Johnson, D. (1976). Changes in nursing students' stereotypic attitudes toward old people. *Nursing Research, 25*, 430–432.

Wolanin, M. (1983). Scope of the problem and its diagnosis. *Geriatric Nursing, 4*(4), 227–230.

Wolanin, M., & Phillips, L. (1981). *Confusion: Prevention and care.* St. Louis: Mosby.

13

Nutrition

COMPONENTS OF ADEQUATE NUTRITION IN ELDERS

Older persons need fewer calories. Recommended daily caloric intake for a man age 51–75 is 2400 calories. Recommended caloric intake for women age 51–75 is 1800 calories. As age increases, caloric requirements decrease. Recommended daily caloric intake for a man over age 75 is 2050 calories. Recommended daily caloric intake for a woman over age 75 is 1600 calories a day (Johnson & Pawlson, 1981, p. 304).

About 1 g of protein per kg of body weight is required for maintenance of body systems. For an older person, 10% to 12% of total caloric intake should come from protein. Carbohydrate intake should be 80% of the total caloric intake. Fat intake should be 10% of the total daily caloric intake according to Pritiken and Cisney (1986, p. 181).

However, illnesses, both acute and chronic, and injury alter nutritional requirements. Additional calories and protein are required for repair and maintenance of body systems during illness and disease.

Major sources of protein are meat, fish, eggs, 2% or skim milk, and low-fat milk products. Major sources of carbohydrate are sugars and starches, including those found in grains, fruits, and vegetables. The carbohydrate intake of older persons should be predominately from cereals, fruits, and vegetables. Major sources of fat are animal fats, butter, and plant oils. The relationship between fat intake and atherosclerosis remains controversial. Research is lacking to either support or refute the need for a fat-modified or cholesterol-lowering diet for the older person (McGandy, 1986).

In addition to protein, carbohydrates, and fats, attention must be paid to vitamin and mineral content of the diets of older persons. A very significant mineral in the diets of older persons is calcium. There is a definite relationship between osteoporosis and low calcium intake (Trollinger, Dowhler, & Calin, 1981, p. 218). Debilitated persons are at greatest risk for developing accelerated osteoporosis. According to Yen (1986), postmenopausal women who are not taking estrogen need 1500 mg of calcium a day to help prevent osteoporosis, while postmenopausal women who take estrogen need 1000 mg of calcium per day. Additionally, Bailey and Certa (1986) state that in addition to decreased calcium intake, absorption efficiency also declines with age. Foods high in calcium include dairy products and vegetables, especially collard greens, turnip greens, and kale.

Iron deficiency anemia is also very prevalent among older persons. Older persons should have 10 mg of iron daily. This is equivalent to at least 4 oz of meat daily.

Vitamin C, or ascorbic acid, is another important dietary constituent. Citrus fruits are the major source of vitamin C, which is also important in the utilization of other vitamins. Zinc, which is abundantly present in green vegetables, effects the acuity of the sense of taste. Although there are age-associated decreases in the number of taste buds, an adequate amount of zinc in the diet can prevent acceleration of the loss of taste (Dickman, 1979, p. 82).

Fiber is another important dietary consideration for older persons. Fiber is very helpful in preventing constipation, which is often a problem of elders. The most economical source of fiber is raw bran, often called miller's bran. This product may be added to hot cereals or other foods and is quite palatable. Certain cereals, including *All-Bran*™, *Fiber One*™, and *Bran Buds*™ are also high in fiber. Fruits and vegetables are sources of fiber and an important part of a balanced diet.

An adequate fluid intake is also an important part of the daily diet. Older persons should have a fluid intake of at least 2 L/day, if not contraindicated (Dickman, 1979, p. 82). Fluids should be given throughout the day and should be readily accessible to the older person.

PROMOTING SOUND NUTRITION

Although older persons require fewer calories, they are at risk to develop malnutrition for a variety of reasons. Older persons living at home simply may not have enough energy to prepare their meals. The persons may not be able to accomplish cooking due to alterations in physical mobility or alterations in vision. It is important to assess the older person's ability to see and taste food. This is particularly important in the home. Older persons may be unable to see or smell spoiled food.

Additionally, older persons may not be able to accomplish shopping and marketing. Many older persons do not drive; grocery stores are seldom located in residential neighborhoods, and public transportation is often unavailable. Older persons may also have difficulty managing large shopping bags from the grocery stores. Such persons can be referred to congregate meal programs or Meals-on-Wheels. In some communities shopping services and/or transportation services are available.

Older persons who live in residential hotels may not have access to full cooking, refrigeration, or food storage facilities. They frequently rely on prepackaged "instant" foods that are high in sodium and saturated fat.

The cost of fresh meats, fruits, and vegetables may be prohibitive for older persons on fixed incomes. Such persons may be eligible for economic assistance programs such as food stamps. Food is also frequently packaged in portions or containers that are too large for one or two. Older persons may be reluctant to spend money on items that might be wasted.

Finally, if the person lives alone there may be no motivation to cook due to solitude and loneliness. Due to the lack of someone to share meals with, the person is prone to develop the "tea and toast" syndrome. Older men who have become widowers may not know how to cook or may be unaware of the components of proper nutrition.

Inadequate nutrition is not limited to older persons who live at home. In acute care facilities persons often receive nothing by mouth after surgery or in preparation for diagnostic tests that also require bowel purging. In long term care facilities there are often numerous people who need assistance with eating; staff members may be hurried or may have to feed several persons at once. Choking frequently occurs when a person is fed too fast; choking not only presents an imminent danger to life, but also creates fear and reluctance to eat.

A nutritional assessment must examine both psychosocial and physical parameters. Moehrlin, Wolanin, and Burnside (1981, p. 332–333) recommend that those who live alone, those on low income, those with recent bereavement, those who abuse alcohol, and those who are confused be considered as high risk for developing malnutrition. Such persons should be referred to a qualified dietician.

The most nutritionally sound diet in the world is of no value unless the person is able to eat the food presented. Caregivers must give special attention to the ability of older persons to feed themselves, and to chew and swallow foods. Many debilitating conditions, such as stroke and arthritis, may limit self-feeding ability. Caregivers should also give attention to the ability of older persons to see their food. It is often helpful to use colored dishes to provide contrast and to reduce glare. Certain physical conditions, such as glaucoma, cataracts, and visual changes associated with stroke, may prevent an older person from seeing the food.

Dishes must be positioned with disabilities in mind. The food should be placed in front of the person, and the person should be seated in a chair whenever possible and the caregiver should talk to the person being fed. The person must be told what food he is eating. If an older person requires assistance with eating, the caregiver must not rush or hurry the feeding process. The person should be positioned as upright as possible to facilitate swallowing and stomach filling.

The condition of the mouth and teeth is one of the most important considerations in the ability of older persons to eat. Teeth that are in poor condition and periodontal disease may interfere with the ability to chew and swallow. Eating may actually be painful if these conditions are present. It may be necessary to chop or puree foods if they cannot be chewed.

Ill-fitting dentures also may cause difficulty in chewing and swallowing, or increase the possibility of contracting or exacerbating periodontal disease. Dentures can often be adjusted, or special denture liners can be used to correct dentures that fit poorly.

Good oral hygiene must be maintained. Cleaning the teeth and mouth is best done with a brush with soft bristles. Special attention must be given to denture cleaning after meals, since food may become trapped between the teeth or impacted under the denture.

Medication should not be added to food at mealtime unless the medication is prescribed to be administered at mealtime. Many medications interfere with the assimilation of nutrients, and some foods interfere with the assimilation of medication. When it is necessary to administer medication with food to increase palatability or acceptance, the pharmacist should be consulted to avoid possible food–drug interaction.

Guidance for an older person to maintain and promote better nutritional health requires that the caregiver is knowledgeable about nutrition. Cultural, economic, and psychosocial factors influence the eating behavior of the older person. The caregiver must have an understanding of these factors and ability to use the information when counseling the elderly. The caregiver must also be aware of programs and resources available to help meet food and nutrition needs. Recognition of persons who might benefit from nutritional assessment or counseling and referral to appropriate resources is an important aspect of nursing practice.

LEARNING CHECK

1. As age increases, caloric requirements _____ .
2. Additional calories are needed during _____ and _____ .
3. There is a relationship between low calcium intake and _____ .
4. The sense of taste is enhanced by _____ .
5. Constipation is often relieved by the addition of _____ to the diet.
6. _____ should not be added to food.
7. Factors that influence the eating behavior of the older person are _____ , _____ , and _____ .
8. The caregiver must be aware of _____ and _____ to help meet nutritional needs.
9. Older persons living alone may not eat properly due to _____ .

REFERENCES

Bailey, L. B., & Certa, J.J. (1986). Diagnoses and treatment of nutritional disorders in older patients. *Geriatrics, 39*(8), 67–74.

Dickman, S. R. (1979). Nutritional needs and effects of poor nutrition in elderly persons. In A. M. Reinhart and M. Quinn (Eds.), *Current practice in gerontological nursing*. St. Louis: Mosby.

Johnson, J., & Pawlson, G.L. (1981). Health maintenance. In M. O'Hara-Devereaux, L. H. Andrus, & C. D. Scott (Eds.), *Eldercare*. New York: Grune and Stratton.

McGandy, R. (1986). Role of nutrition in cardiovascular disease over fifty still unclear. *Journal of Gerontologic Nursing, 12*(4), 112.

Moehrlin, B., Wolanin, M.O., & Burnside, I.M. (1981). Nutrition and the elderly. In I. M. Burnside (Ed.), *Nursing and the aged*. New York: McGraw-Hill.

Pritiken, N., & Cisney, N. (1986). Dietary recommendations for older Americans. In K. Dychtwald (Ed.), *Wellness and health promotion for the elderly*. Rockville, MD: Aspen Systems.

Trollinger, J., Dowhler, D., & Calin, A. (1981). Musculoskeletal system. In M. O'Hara-Devereaux, L. H. Andrus, & C. D. Scott (Eds.), *Eldercare*. New York: Grune and Stratton.

Yen, P.K. (1986). Ten tips for teaching. *Geriatric Nursing, 7*(2), 112.

14

The Facilitative Environment

LONG-TERM CARE FACILITY

It is well known that the physical environment influences well-being, learning, and functioning. Environment is always a prime concern in nursery schools and kindergartens; desks, chairs, lighting, toilets, and other equipment are chosen with the physical and developmental characteristics of the children who use them in mind. A youngster is not given a desk or chair that is intended for a high school student. Supplies, such as thick crayons and large print books, are chosen to facilitate the learning and development of the children. A well-planned environment is also critical to facilitate physical functioning and to achieve the psychosocial well-being of older persons in long-term care facilities.

A prime consideration in nursing homes must be the safety of the residents. Many safety regulations are required by local, state, and federal laws, which also control the licensure of these facilities. Water temperature devices, sanitation rules, electrical codes, handrails, and fire alarms are examples of areas of regulations. In addition to the legal regulations, there are numerous other safety considerations. Call bells must be accessible in all areas and must be easy to operate. Floors must have a nonskid finish or texture and be free of clutter and barriers to mobility. Bathrooms, bathtubs, and showers must also have a nonskid surface and have grab bars installed at proper levels to assist in mobility and prevent falls.

It is particularly important to consider the needs of each individual with respect to the environment. For example, if a person has diminished vision or is hemianoptic, the bed should be positioned so the person's "good" side is toward the door, away from the wall. Similarly, overbed tables, clocks, calendars, and water pitchers must be positioned so the person can see them. Beds should be kept in the low position, except when the caregiver is performing direct care activities. Bedrails should also be used at all times to prevent falls. And, of course, the call bell must be accessible at all times.

Chairs and wheelchairs should be properly selected for the older person. Chairs should have arms, and the seat should be at the proper height to avoid extreme hip or knee flexion. Chairs also should have high backs for support of the upper body and head.

While the purpose of wheelchairs is to promote mobility, the seats of many of the collapsible-type wheelchairs are excessively rigid and can lead to compromised circulation when long periods of time are spent in them. Also, collapsible wheelchairs usually do not have high backs for head support. When an older person has decrements in mobility that necessitate the use of a wheelchair, the wheelchair should be regarded as a central part of the person's environment, and considerable attention should be given to its selection and adjustment. Whenever possible, the older persons should have their own wheelchairs marked with their names.

"High-rise" seats, which easily attach to toilet seats, should be used for tall persons and for persons with limited hip flexion to facilitate mobility and toileting.

Providing privacy is also crucial to maintenance of a person's well-being. All persons need "personal space," or their own territory. Residents of long-term care facilities establish their own territories through frequent use. For example, the personal boundary or territory of a person who is bedridden would be limited to the room, if it is a private room; or, if not, to the area surrounding the bed. The older person should be given the choice of placement of personal effects and furniture for the "personal space" whenever possible, and such decisions should be respected by the caregivers. Curtains or movable screens provide privacy and personal space in semi-private rooms. Clocks with large numerals and hands, a calendar, pictures of family and pets, favorite plants, and a favorite chair should be included in the personal space of residents of long-term care facilities.

Careful planning is necessary to transfer a resident to another room. Such moves must be made with the needs of the older person rather than the needs of the caregiver in mind. The older person should be a participant in decisions regarding relocation, and should be allowed to direct and participate in the packing and moving of personal possessions. If it is necessary to transfer an older person to a hospital, at least one item from the person's environment, such as a favorite picture, should be sent along. The caregivers at the receiving institution must be notified of the existence and significance of the object. Such considerations are very helpful in preventing relocation confusion and trauma.

Caregivers should always knock and identify themselves when entering the personal space and territory regardless of the physical or cognitive state of the resident.

Age-associated decrements in function of the special senses have previously been discussed. With advancing age, increased illumination is needed for general vision and reading. Eyes also become more sensitive to glare; therefore, lamp bulbs or illumination devices should be glare free but sufficiently bright. Fluorescent bulbs provide good illumination, but produce intense glare if not adequately screened or shaded. Care must be taken to avoid illumination devices that might become excessively hot and cause burns.

The warm colors (oranges, yellows, reds) are better perceived by the aging person than the cool colors (blues and greens). It is very helpful to have doorways, hallways, or other important places, such as bathrooms, painted with the warm colors to aid in identification. It is also helpful to identify a person's room with the occupant's name in letters 2 to 3 in high on a contrasting background. A picture of the person(s) can also be used on or near the door as an aid to orient the persons as well as visitors and staff. A sense of personal space, as well as identification, can be enhanced with individual door decorations, such as wreaths, artificial flowers, or other unbreakable objects.

While hallways must be barrier free, chairs or benches should be available for resting places in long hallways. Plants can also be used to break up great lengths and provide aesthetic stimulation. Staff members should wear name tags printed in contrasting colors. It is also helpful to have pictures (with names) of staff members displayed in central areas, such as nursing stations.

The hearing of older persons also should be an environmental consideration. Excessive sound can be very stressful, can interfere with rest, and can lead to disorientation. Carpeting, plastic utensils, and handheld (or earpiece) TV/radio sound controls aid in noise reduction. Sound amplification systems that do not interfere with hearing aid function should be used. Soft chimes or other auditory clues may be used to announce meal times or other events.

An older person's tactile sensation is best stimulated through personal touch. Touching is nurturing. Older persons who are touched during conversation respond more positively. The caregiver should assess for individual and cultural factors as to whether the person is open to touch. In the environment, this sense can be enhanced through the use of texturized wall coverings or wall hangings, and special fabrics for clothing. Staff members of occupational therapy or activity departments can use a variety of materials to augment tactile sensation.

The environment of long-term care facilities should be used to maximize the persons' abilities and comfort, while providing security and privacy. As often as possible, input from the residents should be elicited, respected, and acted upon.

HOME ENVIRONMENT

In the home health care setting, assessment of the environment is crucial to the success of the care plan. There are numerous areas that require evaluation, which begins at the entrance to the client's residence. The exterior of the residence should be observed for general exterior condition, maintenance, and the presence of screens and storm windows.

If steps are present, they must be in good repair and of a nonslip surface. Spray-on or self-adherent products to create a nonslip surface are available in hardware and building supply stores. If there are stairs, railings for support must be available and in good repair. Older persons often have alterations in visual perception; stairways must be well lit and glare free. It is often helpful if the treads of the steps or stairs contrast in color to the riser of the stair. Colored tape may be installed at the edge of the stair for added contrast. The client must be able to negotiate the stairs or steps safely. This is especially important if the client has an alteration in mobility or the person has health problems such as respiratory or cardiovascular disease that limit activity. If the client uses a wheelchair, a ramp may be necessary.

The nurse should also observe where the mailbox is located. It should be at a height that is easily accessible to the client, and should be easy to open. Mail slots often are located near the bottom of the door and require bending or stooping to collect the mail. A basket can be attached to the mail slot, or a mailbox can be installed.

Doorways must be easy to open and of adequate width to accommodate assistive devices or wheelchairs. Entrance doors should have locks, preferably a dead bolt variety, to provide security; locks must be easily operable by the older person. The client must be able to hear if someone is at the door; a doorbell or door knocker may be used.

It should also be determined if the person can hear the telephone and has adequate vision to place calls. Bell amplifiers and flashing lights that indicate incoming calls are available from the various telephone companies. Also, large "stick-on" numeral sheets are available from telephone companies or in variety stores. The phone number of emergency services should be placed on the phone. If the client does not have a telephone, the nurse must determine how assistance is summoned. It may be necessary to obtain a device that will automatically summon assistance, or to devise a system for assistance with a neighbor.

Smoke alarms should be present; most communities have local ordinances that require alarms in apartment dwellings and subsidized housing, but smoke alarms may be absent in private homes. The alarm of the detection device must be clearly audible or visible to the client. Most smoke detectors have a safety feature to indicate low battery power; the client must be knowledgeable about this type of indicator. Some communities have programs that provide smoke detectors for free or at a reduced cost to persons who need them.

The adequacy of the heating/cooling system should be evaluated. The home must be warm enough for the client in cool weather and sufficiently cool during periods of hot weather. Air conditioning is often essential for clients who have chronic obstructive pulmonary disease (COPD) or cardiovascular problems. Various governmental agencies provide assistance with home weatherization and repair, and there are also state and county programs that may provide assistance with energy bills.

The interior of the residence should be evaluated for general cleanliness and safety. The floors shoud be free of clutter and throw rugs. It may be necessary to rearrange furniture to provide a barrier-free pathway for the client. Homemaker/chore-type services are generally available through various state and community agencies.

Good illumination is also necessary. Conversion fluorescent light bulbs are relatively inexpensive, easy to install, and helpful for increasing illumination. Extension cords should not be used unless absolutely necessary. If it is necessary to use extension cords, they must be placed behind furniture or secured firmly to the floor with duct tape.

The area for food preparation and storage requires special assessment. Ideally, there should be adequate counter space located at the proper height for the client. The stove should be equipped with controls that the clilent can easily operate. Older persons should be cautioned to avoid wearing bathrobes or loose clothing when cooking since these can easily contact a hot burner and catch fire. Pots and pans, dishes, and utensils should be easily accessible. The refrigerator must be capable of maintaining food at 40 to 45° F. The sink should be equipped with faucets that the client can easily operate.

Unfortunately, many older persons do not reside in optimal housing or have adequate financial resources. The stove may be a hot plate in some area of the home. Such devices should be checked for safety; the cords and plugs must be intact. The use of multiple plug devices to create additional electric outlets should be discouraged. If refrigeration is not available or adequate, an ice chest with long-lasting ice packs may be used. The client may require nutritional support services such as Meals-on-Wheels, or the client can be referred to congregate meal programs.

The bathroom should be equipped with grab bars located by the tub/shower and toilet. Christopher (1986) suggests that the color of the toilet seat and sink contrast with surrounding surfaces. This can be accomplished by the application of colored tape or contact paper. Special toilet seats are available from medical supply firms or catalogs. The bathtub or shower should have a nonslip surface, or have nonslip appliqués or strips installed. A sturdy chair or stool may be used for additional safety in the shower. The use of electrical appliances in the bathroom should be discouraged; these can eaily cause electrical shock or electrocution.

Modification in the sleeping arrangements may have to be implemented if the client has alterations in mobility that preclude reaching a distant bedroom or a bedroom on a different level. The nurse should also determine where the laundry is done. Laundry rooms are frequently located on lower levels of private homes as well as in congregate housing and apartment complexes. The client may not have adequate mobility or energy to accomplish laundry tasks.

Modifications in the environment may be especially necessary if the client has a chronic brain disorder such as Alzheimer's disease. Home care may not be possible unless the client has a spouse or other person who can provide supervision and care. Since persons with chronic brain disorders tend to wander, it is often helpful to put jingle bells on exterior doors. Prillaman and Junk (1984) also recommend that door locks be put near the bottom of the door; the confused person will not readily find the door lock, and security will be maintained. Privacy locks on interior doors should be removed or securely taped. This modification will prevent the confused person from accidentally being locked in a room.

Control knobs of gas stoves may be removed to prevent

potential fires or accidental burns. A master switch may be installed in an inconspicuous place on an electric range. Locks should be installed on cupboards that contain hazardous materials, such as cleaning products. Knives and medicines should be kept in locked boxes or drawers. Items of value, such as jewelry and important documents, should also be kept in a secure place. Glassware and other breakable objects should be kept out of easy reach.

It may be helpful to "color code" the bathroom door in a primary color with paint or contact paper as a memory aid. Confused persons may have great difficulty in choosing apparel if a great many items are available. Only a few favorite items should be left in closets and dresser drawers to reduce confusion.

There are agencies in most counties or communities that can supply hospital beds, commodes, oxygen, and other medical equipment. At this time, Medicare (Part B) covers 80% of the cost of certain medical equipment, and Medicaid may pay for some equipment. Additionally, certain health-related organizations, such as The American Red Cross and the American Cancer Society, have equipment available for loan or rent at a low cost. Various religious groups, such as St. Vincent de Paul Society and the Lutheran Brotherhood, and veterans' organizations, such as the American Legion and the Veterans of Foreign Wars, also may provide assistance in obtaining equipment or home health supplies.

The findings of the 1981 White House Conference on Aging clearly indicate that older persons desire to remain in their own homes, and that a national commitment should be made to facilitate this wish. A thorough assessment of the home environment, coupled with a knowledge of available resources, is an essential component of quality in-home care. The home health nurse has a crucial central role in the provision of a facilitative environment that will enable elders to remain in their homes.

LEARNING CHECK

1. A prime consideration in nursing homes is the _____ of the resident.
2. It is most important to consider the needs of the _____ with respect to the environment.
3. The seats of collapsible wheelchairs can compromise _____ .
4. With advancing age, increased _____ is needed to see.
5. An older person's tactile sensation is best stimulated through the use of _____ _____ .

REFERENCES

Aging in the 80's: Advocacy and action: Final report. (1981). Available from East Central Illinois Area Agency on Aging, 1003 Maplehill Road, Bloomington, IL, 61701.

Christopher, M.A. (1986). Home care for the elderly. *Nursing 86, 16*(7), 50–55.

Prillaman, P., & Junk, R. (1984). *Alzheimer's disease: What you need to know*. Available from the Central Illinois Chapter of the ADRDA, 807 N. Main St., Bloomington, IL, 61701.

PART IV

Refining a Plan of Care

The purposes of Part IV are to:

1. *Formulate nursing diagnoses, nursing goals, and nursing actions of the nursing care plan in various health care settings*
2. *Evaluate the nursing care plan objectively and accurately*
3. *Discuss quality assurance in relation to gerontological nursing practice*
4. *Discuss the multidisciplinary team approach to care planning*
5. *Facilitate the application of the nursing process through selected case studies and learning vignettes in various health care settings*

15

Formulating and Following Up on a Plan of Care

NURSING PLAN OF CARE

The foundation of nursing practice lies in the application of the nursing process in day-to-day care. According to Gordon (1982), the nursing process includes the following components: assessment, diagnosis, planning, intervention, and evaluation. The importance of an adequate assessment is discussed in Chapter 2. While nursing diagnosis is not a new concept, precise taxonomy and language are only now evolving from the National Conferences of Classification of Nursing Diagnosis.

The authors believe that the use of nursing diagnosis is the best method of focusing on the actual or potential health problem(s) of the client. Nursing diagnosis facilitates communication between nurses; discourages "wastebasket" or inaccurate terminology; facilitates communication between nursing and others, including third-party payers; and increases individual accountability.

The problem–etiology–signs/symptoms (PES) method of writing nursing diagnoses is espoused by Gordon (1982). This format suggests a problem statement in concise terms that leads to identification of nursing goals and nursing interventions. The format is useful because the nursing interventions are determined easily by stating the etiology of the health problem. The statement of the etiology must be amenable to nursing practice. Examples of nursing diagnoses, goals, and interventions for various health problems are described in Part II, "Actual or Potential Health Problems of Older Persons."

The key to effective delivery of nursing services is a *written* plan of care that reflects the health problems and needs of the older person. The plan of care is based on data obtained through accurate assessment. Participation of the client is imperative for planning and providing quality nursing care. Nurses have established standards of gerontological practice by which to measure the quality of nursing care. Thus the nurse is responsible and accountable to the recipient of his/her services. It is essential that the nurse has knowledge of the standards in order to achieve high quality practice. The standards of gerontological nursing practice are given in Appendix A.

The plan of care is individualized, specific, *goal-oriented*, and derived from the nursing diagnoses. A goal is the eventual outcome of a health problem that the nurse and the client/patient hope to attain. Short-term goals usually are those that may be achieved within a brief period. Long-term goals are those statements of the desired results of the nursing care. The formulation of these goals serves as the basis for discharge planning and evaluation of nursing care. The nurse is referred to Little and Carnevali (1981) for a more complete discussion of the components and techniques of goal statements.

EVALUATION AND QUALITY ASSURANCE

Evaluation and quality assurance of nursing care reflect the completion or lack of completion of the nursing process. Were the nursing interventions successful, and were the goals achieved?

Evaluation

Evaluation is the component of the nursing process that judges the validity of the nursing diagnoses and effectiveness of the nursing interventions. Evaluation may lead to a decision that the assessment, nursing diagnoses, and subsequent interventions were accurate and appropriate. On the other hand, evaluation may lead to the conclusion that the assessment, diagnoses, or interventions were inaccurate, and that revision is required.

An example of an evaluation resulting in the decision of accuracy of nursing diagnosis is the following:

> After establishment of the nursing diagnoses of potential impairment of skin integrity due to immobility/bedrest, nursing interventions ordered included skin cleansing/lubrication protocols, and repositioning schedules. These interventions were documented in the resident's chart. The resident did not develop any pressure sores; hence, the nursing diagnosis and interventions were accurate and valid.

An example of evaluation resulting in a decision that the assessment and interventions were inaccurate is the following:

> A nursing diagnosis of impaired verbal communication due to cerebrovascular accident was established for a person who spoke only unintelligible phrases after a CVA. Nursing interventions included directions for speaking to the person as well as orders for the use of an assistive communication device. The goal was establishment and maintenance of communication. After one week it was noted that the person continued to use only "garbled" phrases. A careful review of the history revealed that the person did not speak English, but a mid-European language. This was verified after arranging for a visit by a person conversant in the specific language.

> Although the diagnosis of impaired verbal communication was accurate, the etiology was inaccurate. The person was able to

communicate, but not in English. The nursing staff and inter-
preter devised a "word list" for use in communicating with the
person. The original list of nursing interventions was changed.
Communication with the person was finally achieved.

An example of an evaluation which resulted in the decision
that the assessment, nursing diagnosis, and interventions
were inaccurate is the following:

The nursing diagnosis of sleep pattern disturbance due to
stress was formulated when it was observed that an older patient constantly awoke at 4:00 a.m. and was fatigued by 1:00
p.m. The afternoon fatigue interfered with his physical therapy. Nursing interventions included the administration of the
prescribed (prn) hypnotic, the patient's favorite warm beverage
at bedtime, and environment quieting measures. However, the
patient continued to awaken early and his lethargy increased.
    A review of recent literature (Bahr & Gress, 1985) and a review
of the patient's sleep history led to the conclusion that the
pattern of early awakening and the need for an afternoon nap
were normal for the patient. It was postulated that the hypnotic
influenced the increased lethargy. The diagnosis of "decreased
activity tolerance due to fatigue" was formulated. The physical
therapy appointment was rescheduled for later in the afternoon; the patient completed his bath and other morning activities when he awakened at 4:00 a.m. The prn hypnotic was
omitted; the warm beverage continued to be offered. The patient was subsequently able to participate without fatigue in his
therapy and was no longer lethargic.

Evaluation is also an important component of that activity
known as quality assurance, which is mandated by various
licensing and accreditation agencies. Lyon (1983) states that a
concise diagnostic statement defines the outcome desired for
evaluation, audit, and the quality assurance activities.
Hence, the use of nursing diagnosis also simplifies the process of evaluation.

Quality Assurance

Schmadl (1979) defines quality assurance as that activity which assures the consumer of a specified degree of excellence through continuous measurement and evaluation of structural components, goal-directed nursing process, and/or consumer outcome. Preestablished criteria, standards, and available norms are used in the activity.

The most important component of quality assurance is compliance with standards of gerontological nursing practice. Through evaluation it can be determined if:

1. Data have been collected and recorded.
2. Nursing diagnoses have been formulated.
3. A workable plan of care and goals have been developed from the nursing diagnoses.
4. Interventions amenable to nursing practice have been identified and prioritized.
5. The nursing care has been delivered.
6. Collaboration between the client and the nurse has been achieved in the planning and provision of nursing care.

Nurses should welcome the opportunity to serve on quality assurance committees. The importance of evaluation of total care is an integral function of all health care disciplines. The student is referred to suggested nursing care plans of the case studies presented in this chapter.

MULTIDISCIPLINARY PLAN OF CARE

Various regulations require that a multidisciplinary approach be used for care planning in long-term care facilities. The disciplines include, but are not limited to, nursing, medicine, administration, social services, rehabilitative services, and nutrition. The purposes of utilizing this approach are to involve the person in planning his/her care, to clearly delineate goals and responsibilities of each care provider, and to avoid redundancy or omissions in the provison of care. The multidisciplinary approach to care planning and provision begins with the initial interview and assessment, which is described in Chapter 1.

It is most important that the *nursing* plan of care be developed before the multidisciplinary planning conference. By virtue of 24-hour contact with the person, nursing has the most information about the actual and potential needs of the person, and therefore can serve as a guide to other team members in care planning. Collaboration with the multidisciplinary team may result in modification in the nursing plan of care.

CONSIDERATIONS IN HOME HEALTH CARE

Home health care is the most rapidly expanding field of nursing practice, and most home care patients are elderly. Each home care situation is unique and requires complex and multifaceted care. Clients who receive home health care may be discharged to the home following surgery or an illness, a newly diagnosed or chronic health problem, or a terminal illness. Another type of client may be the older person who needs assistance to remain in the home. In these nursing situations, the nurse focuses on prevention of problems and maximizing the client's function. Health care policies are now being developed to enable elderly persons to remain in their own homes, as home care can be efficient and cost-effective in comparison to institutional care.

The home health nurse does not have the advantages of a multidisciplinary team or control of the environment as in the long-term or hospital facilities. Home health care goals include helping the client maintain independence, as well as reaching his or her health potential.

During the initial visit to the home, a biographical data base is begun to obtain health data. Communication techniques are necessary to establish a relationship of trust with the client. The nurse must ask permission to enter the home, unlike in an institutional setting. The client should be informed that all information is confidential. The nurse should early on relate the purpose of the visit and the amount of time that the interview will take. Having identified who the nurse is and what name the client prefers to be called, the nurse is then able to begin a total health assessment. Observation skills are most important in this assessment, as they are throughout the home visit.

It is recommended that the nurse use an assessment instrument to assist in collecting data. The same subjective assessment worksheet that was provided in Chapter 1 may be used in the home. The nurse should, however, choose tools that meet the needs of the particular agency and client.

Assessment of objective data, or the physical examination, begins when the nurse meets the client. The physical assessment worksheet in Chapter 2 is an example of a tool that the nurse may use as a guide through the physical examination, which then completes the total health data base.

Following the comprehensive nursing assessment, the nurse should analyze the data gathered, reach a conclusion about the client's health status, and formulate the nursing diagnoses. Nursing interventions can be developed with the equipment and supplies that the client is familiar with and with which the nurse may improvise.

The nurse must carefully assess the abilities of the client and the caregiver to determine if the most appropriate level of care can be administered in the home. The nurse also serves as an advocate for the client and family. Since the focus of medical practice is often on the management of acute illness, it is not uncommon for physicians to suggest institutionalization without a thorough assessment of the client's capabilities or support systems. It can be the nurse's role to help keep elders in the familiar home environment.

A thorough assessment by the nurse can help determine if the client has adequate capability and support to remain at home. During hospitalization for an acute illness, both the client and the family may be overwhelmed by the amount of supplies and technical expertise required for care and believe that care in the home is not possible. However, it is not always necessary to use expensive or disposable equipment in the home environment. For example, urinary catheters used for intermittent catheterization may be safely cleaned with soap and water and stored in a plastic bag in the home. Similarly, oxygen cannulas and certain suction equipment need not be disposed after each use or within a given time frame. Also, procedures that may appear to be highly technical, such as intravenous or central line infusions, can be taught to the client and/or support persons through one-to-one education and provision of proper resources.

The nurse must assess and respect the wishes of the client and family. In some cases clients may not desire home care and can well afford the cost of a long-term care facility. It has been the experience of the authors that significant numbers of older persons do not regard nursing homes negatively, and in fact have planned for long-term care throughout the years. The authors feel that this belief is principally due to a client's desire not to burden the spouse or family; moreover, this belief may have been mutually agreed upon by the client, spouse, and family members. Also, the authors believe that positive attitudes toward nursing homes often evolve when the client has friends in long-term care facilities, or when the person has had positive experiences with long-term care. The function of the nurse may be to determine if the client is a candidate for home health care, or if an alternative level of care is more congruent with client needs, abilities, and wishes.

Hewner (1986) defined the role of the home care nurse by

asking these nurses: "What is the most important thing you do to help this person stay at home?" Hewner developed 12 empirical groups of nursing interventions; of these, monitoring health status, health teaching, and caregiver support were the categories that nurses used most frequently.

The authors believe that the major role of the nurse in the home care setting is the rapport that exists between the nurse, family, and client. Adaptation of the home environment, education of the caregiver and client, and frequent evaluation of the client's abilities are some of the unique array of services administered to older persons. The support and companionship given by the nurse is the key to success in maintaining clients in the home.

LEARNING CHECK

1. The best method of focusing the actual or potential health problem(s) of the client is the use of _____ _____ .

2. The PES of writing nursing diagnosis means _____ , _____ , _____ .

3. The problem statement leads to identification of nursing _____ and _____ .

4. The statement of the etiology must be _____ to nursing practice.

5. The plan of care is based on data obtained through accurate _____ , and _____ by the client.

6. It is essential that the nurse have knowledge about _____ _____ _____.

7. The plan of care is individualized, specific, and goal oriented, and derived from the _____ _____ .

8. A _____ is the eventual outcome of a health problem that the nurse and client hope to attain.

9. The component of the nursing diagnosis that supports validity of the nursing judgment is _____ .

10. Licensing and accreditation agencies mandate evaluation activities known as _____ .

11. It is most important that the nursing care plan be developed before the _____ planning conference.

12. Nurses must acquire _____ skills as well as _____ skills in order to meet the needs of older persons.

13. A total health data base includes both a _____ and _____ assessment.

14. The _____ assessment represents information collected from the client.

15. The _____ assessment represents information that the nurse collects.

16. Sensitive information is usually collected _____ in the assessment.

17. It is important for the nurse to _____ with the client and family when developing the care plan.

18. A major role of the home health nurse is the _____ that exists between client, family, and nurse.

19. _____ _____ is the most rapidly expanding field of nursing practice.

REFERENCES

Bahr, R. T., Sr., & Gress, L. (1985). The 24-hour cycle: Rhythms of healthy sleep. *Journal of Gerontological Nursing, 11*(4), 14–17.

Gordon, M. (1982) *Nursing diagnosis: Process and application.* New York: McGraw-Hill.

Hewner, S. (1986). Bringing home the health care. *Journal of Gerontological Nursing, 12*(2), 29–35.

Little, D., & Carnevali, D. (1981). *Nursing care planning* (2nd ed.). Philadelphia: Lippincott.

Lyon, B. (1983). *Nursing practice: An exemplification of the statutory definition.* Birmingham, Alabama: Pathway Press.

Schmadl, J. (1979). Quality assurance: Examination of the concept. *Nursing Outlook, 27*(7), 462–465.

16

Selected Case Studies and Learning Vignettes

CASE STUDIES

The following five case studies are designed to demonstrate implementation of the nursing process with older clients receiving nursing care in acute, extended, and home health care facilities. The case studies are organized as in previous chapters using the format of nursing diagnosis and nursing interventions. Examples of goals and discussion of evaluations are also included.

Case Study A

A 91-year-old female is admitted from the emergency room with confusion and dizziness. She is a known diabetic—Type I (IDDM). The laboratory report shows:

Blood glucose: 328 (Normal, 90–120)
Urine: 2+ sugar; acetone, negative

The patient is a widow and lives in her own home in a small rural community.

Nursing Diagnosis #1

Alteration in fluid volume, actual related to inadequate hydration resulting in dry skin and mucous membranes, decreased skin turgor, confusion

Short-term goal: The resolution of altered metabolic state
Long-term goal: Adequate diabetic control at home

Nursing Interventions

1. Monitor blood sugar levels every 4 hours with chem-strips.
2. Administer insulin as ordered.
3. Observe for rapid onset of hypoglycemia as blood sugar drops.
4. Assess skin for turgor and mucous membranes for dryness.
5. Monitor intravenous fluids.
6. Measure intake and output hourly.

Nursing Diagnosis #2

Potential for injury due to confusion and vertigo

Nursing Interventions

1. Maintain safety precautions.
2. Do not restrain.
3. Implement reality orientation measures.
4. Record level of consciousness/orientation hourly.

Nursing Diagnosis #3

Knowledge deficit of management of diabetes

Nursing Interventions

1. Implement diabetic teaching plan.
2. Arrange for nutritionist to visit client.

3. Contact public health nurse for home care.
4. Contact Meals-on-Wheels for special diet at home.

Evaluation

1. Blood sugar maintained at safe level
2. Adequate hydration achieved by measuring intake and output, skin turgor
3. Oriented to time, place, and person
4. A diabetic teaching plan implemented and evaluated
5. Public health nurse, nutritionist, Meals-on-Wheels contacted for home care

Short-term goal is resolved and the long-term goal is in process.

Case Study B

An 87-year-old female is admitted to a long-term care facility following an open-reduction, internal fixation of an intertrochantoric fracture of the left femur. Physical therapy was begun in the acute care hospital, but is progressing slowly due to residual effects of a previous CVA. Activity is limited to transfer from bed to chair for 30 min per day. The patient has an indwelling catheter.

Nursing Diagnosis #1

Impaired physical mobility (Level III) related to restriction of movement resulting in inability to ambulate

Short-term goal: Urinary continence following catheter removal

Long-term goal: Ambulation—resident will walk with assistive device

Nursing Interventions

1. Arrange for physical therapy evaluation.
2. Contact nurse who cared for the resident while in hospital.
3. Conference with physician, physical therapist as soon as possible.
4. Instruct patient in active ROM. Patient to perform active ROM three times per day.
5. Sit patient up in "geri-chair" for meals.

Nursing Diagnosis #2

Potential for impairment of skin integrity due to immobility

Nursing Interventions

1. Assess pressure points daily.
2. Egg-crate mattress on bed.
3. Reposition on a routine schedule, i.e., 11:00 a.m.; 2:00, 4:00, 8:00, 10:00 p.m.

Nursing Diagnosis #3

Potential for urinary infection associated with indwelling catheter

Nursing Interventions

1. Perineal care in a.m. and p.m. using soap and water.
2. Offer at least one glass of fluid every 2 hours.
3. Maintain closed drainage system.
4. Obtain order for discontinuing catheter.

Evaluation

1. Multidisciplinary conference held and ambulation begun
2. Joint mobility maintained
3. Skin integrity maintained

4. Urinary catheter removed with no evidence of infection present

Case Study C

An 83-year-old widower, a former farmer, is a resident of a skilled nursing facility. The resident's medical diagnosis is arteriosclerotic and cerebral vascular disease. A CT scan showed cortical brain atrophy. He is disoriented to person, time, and place. Recently he has refused foods or fluids by "spitting out" anything taken into his mouth. It is thought that he has Alzheimer's disease.

Nursing Diagnosis #1

Alteration in nutrition, less than body requirements due to inability to eat/drink fluids resulting in dry skin and mucous membranes, decreased skin turgor

Short-term goal: Increase oral intake to 2000 cc/24 h

Long-term goal: Prevention of injuries and maintenance of safety measures

Nursing Interventions

1. Maintain accurate records of intake.
2. Attempt 2-week trial of feeding in room.
3. Prior to mealtime:
   a. Lightly stroke around mouth three times with ice cube.
   b. Stroke three times from ear lobe to corner of mouth with ice cube.
   c. Stroke three times along jawbone to center of chin with ice cube.
4. Mealtime:
   a. Give no pureed foods—only chewables.
   b. Present one food at a time.
   c. Use straws with all liquids.
5. Weigh weekly.

Nursing Diagnosis #2

Memory deficit related to perception/cognitive impairment resulting in disorientation

Nursing Interventions

1. Assess and record level of orientation weekly by using MSQ tests.
2. Use name sign on bed.
3. Reminiscence therapy every afternoon:
   a. Discuss past farming activities.
   b. Discuss wife's role in farming.

Nursing Diagnosis #3

Potential for physical injury due to impaired judgment

Nursing Interventions

1. Tape privacy locks.
2. Keep bells that jingle on resident's door.
3. Resident is to wear "memory impaired" bracelet.
4. Safety measures implemented:
   a. Bed in low position.
   b. Siderails up at night.
   c. Remove all glassware.

Evaluation

Oral intake of 2000 cc daily achieved
Resident maintained admission weight
No physical injuries to date
Level of orientation remained about the same as upon admission

Case Study D

A 93-year-old bachelor is admitted to a long-term care facility following discharge from the hospital. The resident understands the medical diagnoses, which include malignant lymphoma and compromised nutritional status. The resident has a Denver-type shunt in place for control of ascites. The resident signed a living will statement prior to hospitalization. Chemotherapy was not recommended due to advanced stage of the malignancy. The resident has a large decubiti on the sacral area. He is very weak, needs to be fed, but is oriented to time, place, and person. He also has an indwelling catheter. He has only distant nieces and nephews. During hospitalization, he constantly expressed a desire to die: "Let me alone, let me die!" and upon admission to the long-term care facility, he made similar statements. Occasionally, the resident complains of generalized pain, which is relieved by parenteral injections.

Nursing Diagnosis #1

Depleted health potential associated with knowledge of terminal disease process and knowledge of impending death, resulting in verbalization of death wish and generalized pain

Short-term goals: 1. Relief of pain
2. Effective nursing management of decubiti
3. Maintenance of hydration

Long-term goal: Resident will be able to verbalize acceptance of impending death and participate in final plans (i.e., funeral, distribution of assets)

Nursing Interventions

1. Explore with resident statements concerning wish to die.
2. Determine how long resident thinks he is going to live.
3. Investigate support systems (e.g., contact nieces, nephews, identify potential friends).
4. Assess spiritual needs—identify clergyman of choice if appropriate.

5. Assess cultural expectations of the dying process (e.g., funeral arrangements).
6. Determine if resident has made appropriate legal arrangements.
7. Investigate possibility for a consultation of the hospice nurse and the resident.

Nursing Diagnosis #2

Alteration in comfort: pain related to knowledge deficit of pain management technique resulting in verbalizations of pain

Nursing Interventions

1. Assess scope of pain ("on a scale of 1 to 10").
2. Titrate medication for pain per physician's order.
3. Investigate other modalities of pain relief (e.g., therapeutic touch, TENS).

Nursing Diagnosis #3

Impairment of skin integrity; actual due to decubiti resulting in open sore on sacral area, 2.5 cm

Nursing Interventions

1. Assess lesions and record every 3 days.
2. Op-site™ protocol:
   a. Cleanse with hydrogen peroxide.
   b. Rinse with sterile water.
   c. Dry with blow dryer on *cool* setting.
3. Use egg-crate mattress.
4. Reposition frequently:
   9:00 and 10:30 a.m.; 12:00, 1:30, 3:00, and 4:30 p.m.

Nursing Diagnosis #4

Alteration in nutrition less than body requirements related to inability to eat and drink resulting in loss of weight, loss of appetite, pale conjunctiva, and dry mucous membranes

Nursing Interventions

1. Place on intake and output and record daily.
2. Contact nutritionist for consultation and evaluation.
3. Determine and provide food and liquid of resident's preference.
4. Weigh weekly on Tuesday.

Evaluation

Resident is pain free without clouding of sensorium. Decubitus ulcer has not progressed—Op-site™ changed per nursing orders. The resident has maintained his baseline weight. Contacts made with potential support system. Nutritional consultation completed. Arrangement for disposition of body made by resident.

Case Study E

The client is a 69-year-old male who was referred to the home health agency from an outpatient clinic. The client has chronic obstructive pulmonary disease (COPD) and a gastric ulcer. He is a retired automotive mechanic. His wife has resided in a nursing home since her cerebrovascular accident and fractured hip. The couple have no children. The client uses public transportation to visit his wife about every 2 weeks. He lives alone in a sparsely appointed low-income apartment complex, which he describes as adequate for his needs. Smoke alarms are present, and the client uses appropriate safety measures such as rubber mats in the shower and deadbolt locks. The client has a telephone, and visits with his next-door neighbor daily.

The client uses the services of a tax-supported medical clinic for his health care. He eats one meal a day at a congregate meal site and has the services of a homemaker for cleaning once a week. He receives Supplemental Social Security, has a small retirement income, and receives Medicare/Medicaid benefits.

The client perceives his health as "not good." His main problem is the inability to "get enough air," and he also describes a history of "blackening out" after "coughing spells" and "shakiness" of his right arm, which causes him to have problems preparing meals. His legs ache when he walks over two blocks. He wishes that he could cease smoking. He reports no allergies and is unsure of his immunization history.

He recently had a physical exam at the outpatient medical facility, which included hearing and vison examinations. He has had numerous hospitalizations because of his COPD. His current medications include: Primatene® mist medihaler, prn; Tagament®, 300mg twice a day; and Restoril®, 15 mg for sleep. The client formerly took an unknown steroid drug for his pulmonary condition.

The client smokes two packages of unfiltered cigarettes a day. He does not drink alcohol. He drinks two cups of caffeinated coffee in the morning.

He reports some deficit in his ability to hear and he wears bifocal eyeglasses. He also states that "food doesn't smell or taste as good as it used to." He attributes this to the large volume cooking done at the congregate meal site.

The client's affect seems somewhat anxious; he is alert and well oriented. Recent and remote memory are intact. The client usually arises at 7:00 a.m. He states, "it takes awhile to get going" because of excessive coughing and sputum production. The client also awakens several times during the night due to coughing. He usually eats Bran Flakes with milk, two doughnuts, and two cups of coffee for breakfast; meat, vegetable, two cups of milk, and bread with butter, fruit, and dessert for lunch; supper consists of a sandwich, jello or pudding, and milk. It is difficult for him to chew because he has only two teeth. He takes no food supplements, and does not receive a therapeutic diet. The client states that his appetite "used to be better." He reports occasional upper abdominal pain, which he attributes to his ulcer.

The client states that he has no problems with urinary incontinence. He is often bothered by constipation, having a hard, brown stool every other day. The usual time of defecation is after breakfast. Much straining is required and he often becomes short of breath.

He has no leisure activities or hobbies. He often sleeps in his recliner and always uses two pillows when he sleeps in bed. He is able to accomplish bathing and grooming independently. He tries to conserve his energy for visiting his wife in the nursing home.

He has shortness of breath, which limits activity, and coughs with copious sputum. Hot humid weather increases his shortness of breath. Although his apartment is air conditioned, he does not have a humidifier for use in the home heating season.

The client wishes that his health was better. He also wishes that he could take care of his wife, or at least have adequate energy to visit her more frequently. He has many financial concerns and fears future medical bills. He is lonely most of the time, but does not have adequate energy for additional social contacts.

Nursing Diagnosis #1

Ineffective airway clearance related to thoracic breathing and chronic smoking

Short-term goal: Practice breathing exercises

Long-term goal: Refer to stop smoking clinic
Increase activity and socialization

Nursing Interventions

1. Provide a developmental environment for learning (i.e., good lighting, quiet, privacy).
2. Explain pathogenesis of emphysema in lay terminology.
3. Demonstrate pursed lip breathing exercises:
    a. Assume a comfortable, upright position.
    b. Inhale through the nose.
    c. Hold breath momentarily.
    d. Exhale through pursed lips in a whistling position.
4. Provide and explain monitoring tool (checklist) of number of times exercises are performed.
5. Obtain means of humidifying air (i.e., boil water on stove).
6. Refer to stop-smoking program or clinic.

Nursing Diagnosis #2

Potential for fluid volume deficit associated with knowledge deficiency related to fluid intake.

Nursing Interventions

1. Instruct on need for 6–8 glasses of fluid daily
2. Determine client's fluid preferences (include jello)
3. Request client to record fluid intake
4. Teach the complications associated with fluid volume deficit:
    a. Metabolic imbalance
    b. Dry skin
    c. Dry bronchial secretions
    d. Excessive fatigue related to coughing dry secretions

Nursing Diagnosis #3

Alteration in nutrition less than body requirements related to inability to prepare, obtain food, poor dentition, and anorexia

Nursing Interventions

1. Refer client to dental services at health agency.
2. Obtain service of home shopping assistance.
3. Provide two meals daily through mobile meals program.
4. Develop list of food preferences.
5. Investigate possible side effect of anorexia related to sleeping medication.

Nursing Diagnosis #4

Sleep pattern disturbance related to coughing episodes, impaired oxygen transport, and lack of exercise

Nursing Interventions

1. Obtain a history of sleep pattern and sleep rituals.
2. Obtain an order for cough medicine to be kept at bedside.
3. Instruct client about relaxation techniques.

Nursing Diagnosis #5

Grieving, dysfunctional, related to impairment of health status of self and wife, and unavailable social support system

Nursing Interventions

1. Positive reinforcement of positive aspects of health status (successes in attaining health goals).
2. Encourage daily phoning to speak with wife and refer to senior transportation service.
3. Refer client to Friendly Visitor program and provide list of available social activities within the apartment complex.

Nursing Diagnosis #6

Potential for injury (trauma) due to falls

Nursing Interventions

1. Install grab bars in shower.
2. Eliminate unsafe throw rugs.
3. Create a barrier-free environment; rearrange furniture if necessary.

Nursing Diagnosis #7

Alteration in elimination: constipation related to lack of exercise and decreased fluid intake

Nursing Interventions

1. Suggest intake of prune and cranberry juices.
2. Instruct sedentary exercises on a daily routine.
3. Increase fluid intake to 6–8 glasses daily.
4. Encourage same-time elimination pattern.

Evaluation

Client has become less short of breath and has enrolled in a stop-smoking program, but has not yet attended classes. A mobile meals service is providing daily meals. The home shopping service is obtaining supplemental groceries for the client. The client reports that he is more rested upon arising. Cough medicine is needed only once during the night. The client is able through the senior transportation program to visit wife more frequently and is participating in one social activity at the apartment complex. The client has not sustained any injury due to falls. Client's constipation problem is resolved.

LEARNING VIGNETTES IN INSTITUTIONAL CARE

The reader is asked to formulate nursing diagnoses and goals from the following client vignettes. The authors have suggested potential diagnoses and goals so that the reader can compare answers, which can be found in Appendix B. It is possible that other correct diagnostic statements and goals may be developed. The vignettes do not include an adequate data base for individualization of the plan of care; therefore the signs/symptoms are not included in the nursing diagnostic statement. The exercise is designed for the identification of actual health problems and the formulation of nursing diagnoses and goals.

Vignette 1

A 65-year-old male has recently entered an intermediate care facility. He retired 6 months ago from his position as president of an engineering firm. His medical diagnoses include Parkinson's disease, osteoarthritis of the lumbar-sacral spine, and hiatal hernia. He has an unsteady gait, and frequently verbalizes the fear of falling. His wife is a nursing instructor at the local university. She visits her husband every day, and is insistent upon participating in her husband's care.

Vignette 2

An 82-year-old housewife is admitted to the hospital. Infiltrating adenocarcinoma of the left breast was diagnosed after an outpatient breast biopsy. Her bone scan was negative. She is scheduled for a mastectomy in the morning. She stated, "What's the use? I'm full of cancer. I don't want to lose my breast!"

Vignette 3

A 78-year-old female retired elementary school teacher has returned to the long-term care facility following an outpatient cataract phacoemulsification/aspiration and lens implant of the right eye. She has a shield in place over the operated right eye. Other medical problems include residual weakness of her left arm and left leg from a CVA, and diabetes mellitus, Type II (NIDDM).

Vignette 4

A 92-year-old male has been a resident in the nursing home for 7 years. He has a permanent colostomy, which requires irrigation. He had a CVA 8 years ago, has weakness in his right arm and leg, and has aphasia. He recently developed incontinence at night. His scrotal and perineal skin is becoming irritated. He is also very hard of hearing and cannot see without his glasses.

LEARNING VIGNETTES IN HOME HEALTH CARE

Vignette 5

The client is a 102-year-old female who resides in her own home with her two widowed daughters, aged 78 and 80. She has had several cerebrovascular accidents and is generally bedfast. She requires total assistance, provided by the daughters, with all activities of daily living. The physician has recently suggested that the daughters consider a nursing home for the mother since "they are getting older." The daughters contacted the home health agency because they were worried that they "weren't taking good care" of their mother. During the initial interview and assessment the daughters expressed their own desires to continue caring for their mother, as well as fulfilling their mother's wish to remain at home. The daughters are in good health, and it was determined that there is excellent support with homemaking and respite care from other family members and church people. It was also determined that the family group was not in financial distress. Assessment of the environment revealed that all equipment necessary for the mother's care was present, and that there were no environmental safety hazards. The mother was found to be in an excellent state of hygiene. The daughters were able to feed, toilet, bathe, and transfer her without difficulty. The home health nurse therefore regarded not the mother, but the daughters, as the clients, and formulated nursing diagnoses.

Vignette 6

The client is an 85-year-old male who was referred to the home health agency by his personal physician. The client was scheduled to have outpatient surgery for removal of a right cataract with a lens implant. Hypokalemia, hypoproteinemia, and iron deficiency anemia were diagnosed through presurgical testing. The surgery was cancelled. The following data was gathered and substantiated during the initial visit:

The client is a bachelor who had recently moved to the community from a large metropolitan area. The reason for his relocation was to be near his next of kin, a niece. The client had lived in the same neighborhood since his emigration from Italy as a child. He had worked as a gardener and laborer, and has a fixed retirement income. The client stated that "all my friends are gone; they are in homes (nursing) or dead," and that the niece and her family are his only contacts. He lives in a two room furnished apartment, which he feels is adequate for his needs. There is a large supermarket within walking distance where he shops.

The nutritional history revealed a diet that lacked essential nutrients. The client did not like to cook, had difficulty reading directions for food preparation, and had difficulty seeing items in the grocery store as well as the dial on the oven control. Except for dinner on Sundays with the niece, his usual meal pattern was instant coffee and doughnuts for breakfast, canned pasta for lunch, and a sandwich from the supermarket's deli for supper. Snacks were packaged cookies and occasional fresh fruit. Milk and vegetables were never consumed.

The client reported that he had not noticed his failing vision until the relocation. He also stated that he felt weak, tired, and was not able to walk farther than two blocks, although he formerly had a great exercise tolerance. He also expressed a fear of falling due to his weakness. The objective assessment by the physician indicated that the client has osteoarthritis in addition to the nutrition imbalance, but no other major health problems.

Vignette 7

The client is a 79-year-old widow who was referred to the home health agency because of noncompliance with her medication regime and for blood pressure monitoring. She had been recently hospitalized because of digitalis toxicity. The client was known to have congestive heart failure and hypertension. The client's medication included Lanoxin, 0.125 mg once a day; Lasix, 20 mg twice a day; Aldomet, 125 mg twice a day; and Kaon, one tablet twice a day.

During the initial visit the client stated, "I just can't remember if I've taken my pills or not." It was determined that the client had adequate support from friends and family members, and that the home was well maintained and safe.

APPENDIX A

American Nurses' Association Standards of Gerontological Nursing Practice

STANDARD I

Data are systematically and continuously collected about the health status of the older adult. The data are accessible, communicated, and recorded.

STANDARD II

Nursing diagnoses are derived from the identified normal responses of the individual to aging and the data collected about the health status of the older adult.

STANDARD III

A plan of nursing care is developed in conjunction with the older adult and/or significant others that includes goals derived from the nursing diagnosis.

From: American Nurses' Association, *Standards of Gerontological Nursing Practice*. Kansas City, MO: American Nurses' Association, 1976. Reprinted with permission.

STANDARD IV

The plan of nursing care includes priorities and prescribed nursing approaches and measures to achieve the goals derived from the nursing diagnosis.

STANDARD V

The plan of care is implemented, using appropriate nursing actions.

STANDARD VI

The older adult and/or significant other(s) participate in determining the process attained in the achievement of established goals.

STANDARD VII

The older adult and/or significant other(s) participate in the ongoing process of assessment, the setting of new goals, the reordering of priorities, the revision of plans for nursing care, and the initiation of new nursing actions.

APPENDIX B

Answers to Learning Checks and Learning Vignettes

LEARNING CHECKS

Chapter 1

1. prior
2. reason for seeking health care; principal health problem
3. medication and nutrition
4. expectations of care
5. terminated
6. before discharge
7. initially; communication; relieving anxiety
8. paraphrase; repeat

Chapter 2

1. elasticity; subcutaneous
2. liver spots
3. respiratory
4. stretch
5. alveoli; bronchioles
6. oxygenation
7. PaO_2
8. stiffer, less compliant
9. systolic; ejection murmurs
10. valves
11. systolic
12. tissue
13. antibodies
14. abrasion
15. peristalsis; motility
16. liver
17. emptying time
18. warm
19. cerumen

20. strength; size
21. cartilages
22. height
23. demineralizes
24. desire; functioning
25. alkaline
26. males; females

27. decreases; increases
28. concentrate
29. capacity; empty
30. prostate
31. amyloid
32. neurotransmitters
33. short-term

Chapter 3

1. Fever
2. splinting
3. humidifier

4. rest
5. pursed-lip
6. oxygen

Chapter 4

1. chest pain
2. Lenegre's disease
3. hypertension
4. sixty
5. nitroglycerin

6. congestive heart failure
7. iron deficiency
8. empty
9. vitamin B_{12}
10. sore tongue

Chapter 5

1. Incontinence
2. cause
3. bladder infection
4. benign prostatic hypertrophy

5. foreskin
6. vaginitis
7. prolapsed uterus

Chapter 6

1. Xerostomia
2. hiatal hernia
3. high fiber

4. gallbladder disease
5. prevention

Chapter 7

1. demineralization
2. osteoarthritis
3. fingertip to fingertip
4. rheumatoid arthritis
5. immobilization

Chapter 8

1. pill-rolling
2. muscle rigidity
3. tardive dyskinesia
4. 24 hours
5. acute; chronic
6. Alzheimer's disease
7. CVA or stroke
8. TIA
9. area of brain; amount of brain tissue involved
10. left side
11. receptive aphasia

Chapter 9

1. peripheral vision
2. blindness
3. read
4. audiometric testing
5. presbycusis

Chapter 10

1. hyperglycemia
2. ketoacidosis
3. increases
4. cold
5. myxedema coma
6. arrhythmia; heart failure

Chapter 11

1. four
2. venous
3. arterial
4. arterial
5. stasis dermatitis

Chapter 12

1. autonomy, independence
2. Stereotyping
3. deindividuation
4. disengagement
5. dementia; depression
6. support system
7. self-esteem

Chapter 13

1. decrease
2. illness; disease
3. osteoporosis
4. zinc
5. fiber, bran
6. medications
7. cultural; economic; psychosocial
8. programs; resources
9. loneliness

Chapter 14

1. safety
2. individual
3. circulation
4. illumination
5. personal touch

Chapter 15

1. nursing process
2. problem; etiology; signs/symptoms
3. goals; interventions
4. amenable
5. assessment; participation
6. standards of gerontologic nursing
7. nursing diagnosis
8. goal
9. evaluation
10. quality assurance
11. multidisciplinary
12. assessment; technical
13. subjective; objective
14. subjective
15. objective
16. later
17. consult
18. rapport
19. home care

SUGGESTED DIAGNOSES AND GOALS FOR LEARNING VIGNETTES

Vignette 1

Diagnoses

1. Impaired physical mobility related to muscle weakness and tremors
2. Potential for injury related to unsteady gait
3. Fear of falling due to unsteady gait
4. Potential for ineffective family coping associated with wife's behavior.

Goals

Short-term: Participation by wife and client in design of nursing care plan

Long-term: Improvement of mobility

Vignette 2

Diagnoses

1. Fear of impending surgery: knowledge deficit related to scope of disease process
2. Fear of impending death related to medical diagnosis of cancer
3. Body image disturbance due to scheduled mastectomy

Goals

Short-term: Client will understand need for surgery

Long-term: Reach to Recovery will visit client before discharge from hospital

Vignette 3

Diagnoses

1. Uncompensated sensory deficit: vision
2. Potential for injury related to visual loss, muscular weakness in left arm and leg
3. Potential fluid volume deficit (hyperglycemia) due to stress of eye surgery

Goals

Short-term: Correct instillation of ophthalmic medication and adequate control of NIDDM
Long-term: Prevention of injury to right eye

Vignette 4

Diagnoses

1. Impairment of skin integrity related to wetness in scrotal and perineal area
2. Alteration in elimination (urinary incontinence)
3. Self-toileting deficit, Level III, related to need for colostomy irrigation
4. Uncompensated sensory deficit: vision
5. Uncompensated sensory deficit: hearing loss
6. Impaired physical mobility due to weakness of right arm and leg
7. Potential for injury, fall, due to visual impairment and impaired mobility

Goals

Short-term: Maintenance of scrotal and perineal skin integrity
Long-term: Compensated sensory deficits

Vignette 5

Diagnoses

1. Effective family coping pattern: ability to care for mother and expressed desire to continue care
2. Communication deficit related to physician's suggestion for mother's institutionalization

Goals

Short-term: Establish communication between family and physician

Long-term: Daughters continue to care for mother in the home

Nursing Interventions

Nursing interventions included positive reinforcement of the daughters' activities, and immediate personal communication with the physician.

Vignette 6

Diagnoses

1. Alteration in nutrition, less than body requirements, related to inability to obtain and prepare food
2. Knowledge deficit of adequate nutrition
3. Sensory-perceptual alteration related to uncompensated vision
4. Cultural deprivation related to recent relocation
5. Impaired physical mobility due to weakness experienced with mobility and fear of falling
6. Potential for injury, trauma due to fall, related to weakness

Goals

Short-term: Establishment of adequate nutrition
Long-term: Compensated vision problem resolved

Nursing Interventions

The immediate intervention was to refer the client to a congregate meal program that provided one hot meal a day.
Transportation to the site was available. The niece was contacted, and she agreed to assist with shopping. Suggested
meal plans and shopping guides in large print were provided. Fluorescent bulbs were installed to augment the lighting
in the apartment. The oven dial was enhanced with a magic
marker at the moderate and warm temperature settings. A
grab bar was installed in the bathroom shower. Furniture was
rearranged to provide a barrier-free environment as well as
potential support when the client felt weak. Range-of-motion
and sedentary exercises were taught. "Talking books" and
Italian opera recordings were obtained from the library.

Vignette 7

Diagnoses

1. Potential for injury, poisoning, related to incorrect self-
   medication
2. Noncompliance with medication regime due to forgetfulness
3. Alteration in tissue perfusion related to increased cardiac
   work load

Goals

Short-term: Institution of method for memory assistance
Long-term: Implementation of activities to conserve ener-
            gy and decrease the cardiac workload

Nursing Interventions

The immediate intervention was to institute a method for memory assistance to facilitate taking the correct medications. A daily calendar was hung on the kitchen wall. Small soufflé cups in two colors, yellow and blue, and an ice cube tray were obtained. It was agreed that the yellow cup would contain the morning drugs, and the blue cup would indicate the evening drugs. The colors were chosen to connote sunrise and sunset. The cups containing the medication dispensed by the nurse were placed in the ice cube tray. The dates were affixed to the wells of the ice cube tray with pressure sensitive dot stickers. It was determined that the client always watched television newscasts at 8 a.m. and 5:30 p.m. It was agreed that the start of these programs would be the cue for taking the medications. A checklist of the medication and times was written on each page of the calendar.

The client's daily activities were reviewed; it was discovered that the client performed a great deal of physical activity in the morning, but little during the remainder of the day. The client and nurse devised a plan of activities to conserve energy and decrease the cardiac workload. The prescribed low sodium diet was reviewed, and a list of foods high in potassium was provided. The client was also taught how to take her pulse, and instructed not to take the Lanoxin if the heart rate was below 60 beats per minute.

Index

the African cereals because of their adaptation to low, short, and erratic rainfall.

In sum, possibly excluding yams in West Africa, wherever rainfall is sufficient, Africans choose to grow the labor-cheaper crops, even replacing old ones with newer, cheaper crops (yams by maize, maize by cassava, cassava by bananas). They are forced to remain with sorghum and millets in wide areas simply because of the peculiarities of African climate and the lack of substitutes.

It is interesting to consider what Africa must have been like before contact with Asia and America introduced all the low-cost crops—cassava, maize and plantains. Because the main crops would have been African cereals and yams, the higher cost of production of food would have had significant effects on states, for example, as we shall see later.

HUNTING AND GATHERING

Before turning to the production of domestic animals, we should take the time to look at a rather uncommon form of production—hunting and gathering—which is nevertheless not unimportant in the total picture of African food production. Very few people in Africa still depend on it for a livelihood, or even depended on it at the beginning of colonialism. Lee (Scudder 1971) estimated that of the approximately 44,000 San in southern Africa in 1963, only about 9000 were still primarily hunters and gatherers, and the Hadza of Tanzania, one of the main hunting and gathering groups outside southern Africa, who were up to recent times dependent on that mode of production, were few in number. Such people, in fact, depended more on plants than animals for food. The women were the main gatherers therefore they were the main food producers, just as in agriculturally based societies. Scudder (1971) points out that although many, perhaps most, Africans barely engage in hunting and gathering at all, it is an important supplementary source of food, especially during times of famine and the period of seasonal hunger that occurs in the two months or so before harvest in many societies. Some Pokot pastoralists, for example, endure a seasonal hunger period, but the Turu do not, although both would suffer from famine in occasional years. On the other hand, the Tonga of Zambia, whom Scudder studied, regularly depend on gathering in addition to agriculture so that one could speak of them as having a hunting and gathering plus agricultural economy.

The economics of all this have not been carefully examined, but it is possible to guess what they might be. Beginning with pure hunting and gathering, it should first be understood that Africans, unlike ourselves perhaps, do not engage in agriculture because it is more progressive but because ordinarily it is more profitable than other alternatives open to them. Similarly, they abandon agriculture for livestock if they can because compared to agriculture, it is more profitable. If there are some people who still gather, like the San and Hadza, it is probably because in the circumstances, it makes more sense. As long as the San population is small relative to the supply of natural foods there is not much competition for available foods and they actually produce more than agriculturalists, having ample supplies and no seasonal hunger. Yet the steady decline in numbers of gatherers in the last century suggests that among the San, some new elements have entered the picture, upsetting the balance and causing gathering to decline.

Similarly, it is easy to guess that agriculturalists and pastoralists vary in the degree to which they resort to gathering in nonfamine (or even famine) times, dependent on cost relative to return. The Gwembe Tonga, for example, live in a habitat (Zambezi Valley) unusually rich in natural food plants and balanced against population density, probably find the return on expenditure of labor high. For other agriculturalists in more densely populated areas with few natural food plants, the cost of producing a pound of such food is higher than the cost of just enduring hunger for a while or, in the case of pastoralists, selling livestock to buy grain. Furthermore, since return on such labor could be expected to decline at the margin (each additional hour spent leading to less food produced), each society probably will exploit such resources only up to a certain point. The Pokot do gather during the seasonal hunger period thereby saving the necessity of selling livestock, but they will sell during famines when hunger endangers their lives. The Pokot do not exploit their natural resources very extensively probably because they feel that this is time poorly spent compared to inputs into agriculture and animal herding. The Turu scarcely gather or hunt at all. The main relish for their daily porridge is a wild, succulent grass that grows everywhere around a village and requires only a few minutes to gather. They will not fish even where huge catfish or perch are easily obtainable. This compares with their eschewing of pottery, basketry, and other goods manufacture which is also time poorly spent. Again, then, as with various crops, the resultant food produced and its market value is compared with labor costs or opportunity costs of putting their time into other activities. The economic formula varies from place to place because profitability varies from place to place and from time to time.

DOMESTIC ANIMALS

Wherever domestic animals can be raised in Africa, they have important effects on production. The domestic animals of Africa can be ranked in order of value as generally seen by Africans themselves.

Horses are probably the most valuable animals, but they have a very limited distribution (notably in the western sudan), and little is known about them. Therefore we will leave the question of horses aside and turn to camels which are the most valuable beside horses. Camels also have a limited distribution (see Map 3.1), but they are far more common than horses. They are limited principally by the fact that they are adapted to a narrow ecological zone, the desert margins with little water. They are found in most arid places, the fringe of the Sahara in the western sudan, in northeast Africa in the Horn, and in parts of Ethiopia, Kenya, and Sudan. The Somalis are almost entirely camel herders, but the Turkana of northwest Kenya and the Rendille of northern Kenya, to name only two, combine camels with cattle, favoring the latter.

Next to camels in value and far more widely spread and numerous are cattle. There are a number of varieties of cattle in Africa including the Ndama, dwarf cattle in the tsetse-fly zone of West Africa, and the Sanga, long-horned varieties, especially to be found among the Ankole people of western Uganda. The most widespread are the Zebu, humped cattle resembling the Indian Brahmans but smaller and more varied in color. Zebu are hearty animals, able to stand drought and other adverse conditions, but they are poor milk and meat producers, compared to most European type animals. Cattle may be found dispersed over wide areas of Africa (Map 3.2). Except for the small numbers of Ndama of West Africa, they are always in savannah areas. They occur in large numbers in the western sudan, throughout the savannah regions of East Africa (southern Sudan, Ethiopia, Somalia, Kenya, Uganda, Tanzania), and they are found in large numbers in southern Africa from the southern margin of Zambia through Botswana, Zimbabwe-Rhodesia, and South Africa, as well as in Namibia and Angola. Their distribution, in fact, is limited mainly by the tsetse fly (see Map 3.3).

Lack of water reduces the number of cattle to be found in the Kalahari Desert in Botswana, an area which is not desert in the literal sense, but a huge savannah area where the rainfall is so low that domestic animals cannot survive without modern technology to provide wells. Similarly, large parts of East Africa are closed to them because of the water shortage; these areas are left to the camels. Furthermore, shortage of water limits their distribution outside the tsetse zones in West Africa.

Ratios of Cattle to People

The degree of concentration of the animals relative to human population, often expressed as a ratio, has enormous significance for social structure. It has been determined in East Africa that social structures are radically affected when the ratio of cattle to people reaches one cow or more per person (Schneider 1979).

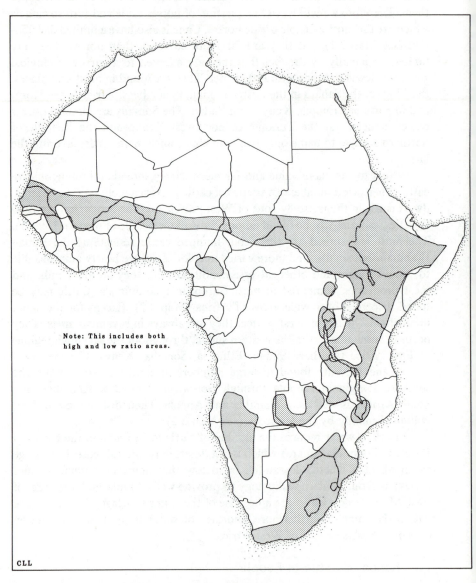

Note: This includes both high and low ratio areas.

CLL

MAP 3.2   Main Cattle Producing Areas
(from Konnerup, 1966)

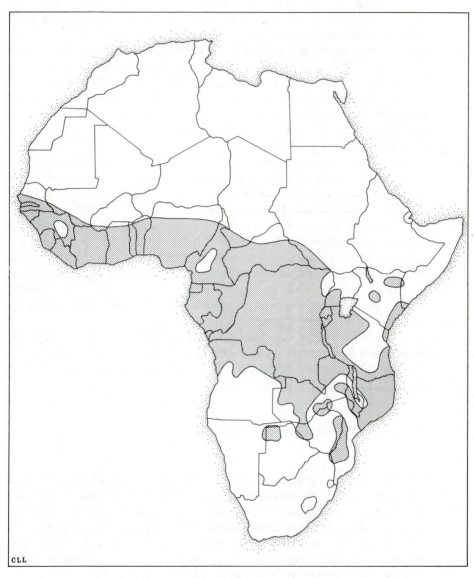

MAP 3.3   Distribution of Tsetse Fly in Africa
(from Konnerup, 1966)

There are only a few places in Africa where this ratio is achieved, a fact not shown in Map 3.2. For example, in northern Nigeria and Niger as well as in Mali, there are sometimes large ratios of cattle to people, especially among the pastoral Fulani, as there are in East Africa, in the southern Sudan, much of Kenya, and parts of western Uganda and north central Tanzania, among such people as the Maasai, Turkana, Somali, Nandi, and Kipsigis, to name a few. In southern Africa these high ratios are found among the Batswana, or Tswana, of Botswana and the Zulu. Low ratios are found in most of Angola, among the Ovimbundu and Ambo, and among the Banyarwanda, or Rwanda, and Banyarundi, or Rundi, north of Lake Tanganyika, as well as in much of the western sudan. For reasons which I shall go into later, I will use the term *pastoral people* only when there are ratios of cattle to people of one-to-one or more, even if these people also raise crops, as most do. Those with lower ratios will be excluded from the classification even though the presence of lower numbers of cattle among them also has an effect on their social systems.

Goats and sheep are the next most valuable animals. In East Africa they are generally treated together, and in fact they look much alike, the sheep having hair rather than wool. Their distribution follows that of cattle, except that goats have a somewhat wider distribution and so are available in small numbers to people in the rain forest zones. Goats and sheep everywhere provide an important source of protein and are slaughtered more readily for food than either cattle or camels.

Chickens are the last domestic animals of value, although dogs are sometimes trained for hunting and are important in some places. Chickens are often used for sacrifices in the rain forest zones and are also important as a source of protein.

Cost of Producing Livestock

The effect of domestic animals on the cost of production may be indicated in the following way. The cost of producing cattle, the most widespread of the valuable large domesticates, is far below the cost of producing crops of equivalent value while the return is much higher. This is due to the fact that Africans value domestic animals much more highly and constantly than crops, just as we value gold. African cattle are not raised as we raise cattle, with extensive housing and expensive feed. At most, they are usually kept out-of-doors, within a cheaply constructed pen, and they are normally not provided with fodder but are taken out to graze. Large numbers of these valuable animals can be tended by a few herdsmen, and they reproduce themselves with little help from their owners.

Cattle and other domestic animals, then, are very valuable, but they are produced with comparatively little labor or capital. It is therefore most practical for African producers to place their emphasis on the production of cattle, camels, sheep, and goats at the expense of domestic crops, if necessary, since the normally high demand for domestic animals insures that food can always be purchased with them. Wherever the production of crops can be combined with the raising of livestock, this will be done, and some Africans, like the Kipsigis of Kenya, raise large amounts of maize while also keeping large herds. If crop production must be forsaken for the benefit of the herds, crops will be abandoned. For example, the northern Somalis raise no crops and herd only camels, and the Turkana raise only a small amount of grain because their marginal, low rainfall habitat, while good for cattle, is poor for crop raising. It even seems possible that the reason more cassava is not grown in livestock-producing areas is that its appeal to goats would require a choice between the two and the decision would inevitably be abandonment of cassava.

Thus while cattle and camels are raised wherever they can be, the effects of possession of herds on social structure is variable and has its greatest impact when the ratio of cattle (or camel equivalents) to people is one cow to a person or more. Only in northeast and southeast Africa are these high ratios possible on a large scale. However, the effect, as we shall see, is mitigated in southeast Africa by long contact with the Europeans who moved into the Cape in the seventeenth century and by the general introduction of ox plowing into the high cattle areas during the last hundred years.

As a result of these facts, we may now introduce a modified model, comparable to the earlier one, which shows the production costs of various products as they progress from highest to lowest in terms of labor:

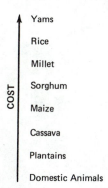

Ordinarily where Africans are producers of large domestics, they also have high labor costs for production of crops since the crops which are compatible with herding are the grains. However, herders also are best able to afford those high labor costs since domestic animal raising is a high-return occupation.

Economically speaking the importance of the fact that all Africans who can raise domestic animals do so because they are repositories of value under-scores the fact that Africans are not just subsistence producers or provisioners. They create goods for trade. Domestic animals raised as repositories of wealth would not make much sense if the producers never traded them. They represent stored up value which can at any time be converted into desirable goods available from others. Grain and other crops can always be bought with domestic animals, as can the service of wives for the production of crops and children. Crops, however, are not always exchangeable for other goods.

THE PRODUCTION OF OTHER GOODS

Africans create a wide variety of goods other than crops and animals, many of which are traded in the regular markets that occur in many places or on a more informal basis. West Africa seems to have been the most highly produc-

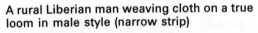

A rural Liberian man weaving cloth on a true loom in male style (narrow strip)

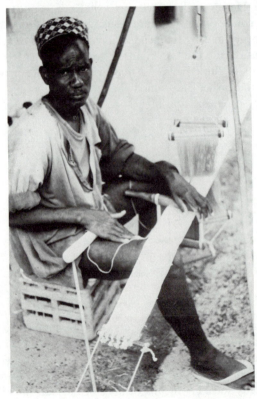

tive of all kinds of goods as was the western Zaire Basin, to judge by the presence there of regular and widespread markets. Vansina's study of production and marketing activities of the Kuba in the 1950s gives an idea of the kinds of products that could be expected in that area: mortars and pestles for processing food products; gourd containers of various shapes and sizes for different purposes; baskets of many varieties for winnowing, carrying cut grain, and so on; firewood; charcoal; carved wooden containers of various shapes and sizes for different purposes; furniture, including benches, stools, beds; skins shaped as bags, clothing, and so on; clay pots of different shapes and sizes; utensils of carved wood; tobacco pipes; awls; cloth made of raffia; iron tools of various types, including knives, hoe heads, axes; raffia ropes; bracelets and other adornments including hats of office; bows and arrows; spears; carved troughs; machetes; wild animal skins, such as the Colobus monkey. The thing to note about this incomplete list is the wide variety of manufactured products needed by African people, a situation which contributes to the growth of exchanges between them and to the existence of marketplaces in some areas, since it would be uneconomical and often impossible for a single household to produce all these things for itself.

PRODUCTION REGIONS OF AFRICA

To conclude this discussion of African production, there is value in summarizing some of the facts (Map 3.4).

West African Region

The main crops are yams and cassava, the first high and the second low in labor cost. This region, with the highest population concentration in Africa, also relies more on root crops than does any other area in the world. The region also contains the highest specialization of production of material goods and, along with that, more intensive periodic market activity. However, it is essentially without large domestic livestock which makes the production of material wealth dependent on manufacturing rather than on breeding.

Rice Region

Though part of the coast is a high rainfall area, this rather small region is unique in its concentration on rice as a main crop. Thus it is an area of very

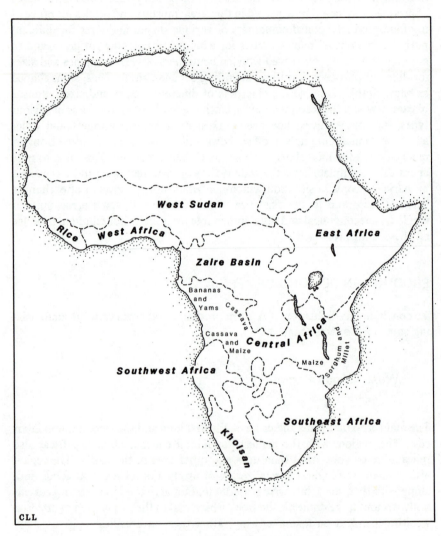

MAP 3.4 Production Regions of Africa

high labor cost. Marketing is less intense than in the rest of the coast, and it is essentially without large domestic livestock. Rice appears to dominate here because it fits a unique ecozone, high in rainfall but without other conditions that would favor yams and cassava, as in the rest of the high rainfall areas to the east.

Zaire Basin

Unlike the West African rain forest, this area is relatively lightly populated and mainly dependent on cassava or, in some places, bananas, making it a low labor cost area. Repositories of value and media of exchange reflect (or reflected) the type of production and include copper, iron, slaves, dogs, chickens, goats, and raffia cloth. The area is without large domestic animals. There is a mixed pattern of periodic markets which are most common in the western part.

Central Africa

While the area originally seems to have been dominated by African cereals, making it a high labor cost area, today this is true only in most of the eastern part, the other parts having been penetrated variously by lower cost crops: bananas, in the far northwest; cassava, in the northwest, outside the banana zone; cassava and maize, in the west, and maize, in a portion of the east. Although this is a low rainfall savannah territory, it is infested with the tsetse fly, just like the rain forests, and so no large domestic animals can be kept. In addition, it is an area of very poor soil in most places, low in fertility even after long fallowing, requiring labor expensive chitemene and other types of crop production methods (including mulching and composting) even in the western cassava areas. The extraordinary methods used to add fertility to the soil and the consequent unusually high labor costs have had a marked effect on the social structure, notably through converting this to a "matrilineal belt" and by creating a high incidence of slavery.

East Africa

Dominant crops in East Africa are African cereals and maize in some places, with plantains in a few select areas, notably Buganda, whose economy is built on them. The area is particularly noted in its eastern part as one with the highest concentration of cattle, and in some places camels, relative to people, equaled only by southern Africa.

Southern Africa

Dominant crops are the African cereals but maize intrudes significantly in the southeastern areas where there is more rainfall. However, like East Africa, this is an area in which high ratios of cattle to people are to be found. Nevertheless, the area has been so affected by European influence, especially with respect to the introduction of trade and ox plowing, that compared to East Africa, important alterations in social structure have resulted.

Southwest Africa

This area might best be included with southern Africa, except for the absence of plows; this allies it more closely with East Africa or the western Sudan. Cattle are important but occur in high ratios only among the Herero. The rest of the area is low ratio and dominated by African cereals or cassava, except among the Herero who raise no crops.

Western Sudan

Because of the presence of cattle in appreciable numbers, this area is similar to East Africa, but it does not have such high ratios, except among some of the Fulani. It is therefore best thought of as an area of low ratio cattle to people with great dependence on labor costly African cereals.

Khoi-San

This is the arid or semiarid Kalahari and Cape Zone. In the past it would have been characterized as containing two types of production, hunting and gathering among the San and cattle raising without agriculture among the Khoi, or Hottentots. In fact, it would have been grouped with the Herero and other Southwest Africans, except for differences in racial type. However, the Khoi,

whose habitat was mainly the better-watered Cape, have long since disappeared, leaving only the San. Their mode of production, depending heavily on
gathering such things as mongongo nuts and hunting, is not readily characterized in terms of cost compared to other African techniques. Lee's work among
the !Kung (Lee 1969) showed, paradoxically, that their food production system, at least the gathering of nuts, was so highly productive that they had to
spend only one-third of their time on food production. Whether this is true
of other kinds of San is not clear.

MARKETS

Turning now to exchange, as most prolific in the production of goods of all
types, West Africa has also developed the most complex forms of production
activities, including guilds of mask makers, carvers, iron workers, dyers and
weavers, and brass casters, to name only some. This has also led to the rise
of complex market systems, with marketplaces occurring at regular intervals,
as seen on Map 3.5 (Smith 1971). The frequency with which markets occur
may be taken as proportional to the amount of goods available and the density
of population. The existence of periodic markets in West Africa varies closely
with the density of population, which is highest in the southern Nigerian area.

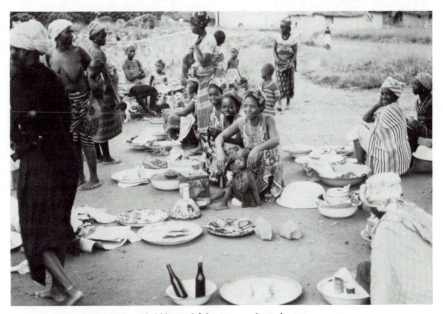

A West African marketplace

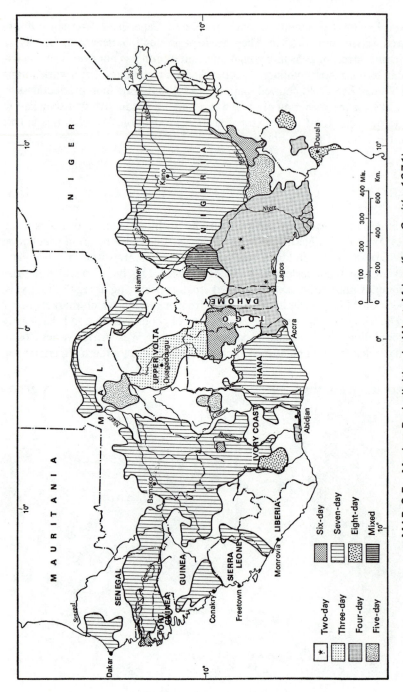

MAP 3.5   Market Periodicities in West Africa *(from Smith, 1971)*

Whereas markets every seventh day are the most common in western West Africa, in southwest Nigeria, the home of the great Yoruba people, they occur every four days or every three days around Ouagadougu, the center of the Mossi empire. Focusing more closely on the Yoruba, Map 3.6 of major Yoruba markets (Morgan and Pugh 1973, 35) shows them as they were in 1886. As is apparent, there is a kind of geometry to the pattern which suggests that the market system of the Yoruba conformed to a theory about the origin of market systems called Central Place Theory. *Central Place Theory* hypothesizes that the spatial relationship of markets and their relative sizes is a product of the market value of the traded goods relative to the cost of transporting them to market. If a Yoruba has something to sell, such as a knife, he will calculate the cost of taking it to market relative to what he expects to get. If he expects to get little, he won't want to take it very far, and if he expects a lot, he is willing to go far. Furthermore, it goes without saying, he will go to the nearest market that will minimize his costs. The result of this situation is that the market system grows geometrically, with different levels of activity and periodicity, the geometric pattern being skewed, however, by the nature of the terrain (rivers to cross, hills to climb).

Bascom (1969, 25) tells us something of the nature of these Yoruba markets:

The markets are composed of areas occupied by women selling the same commodities: poultry in basket coops, tethered goats and sheep, yams, peppers, plantains, green vegetables, meat, salt, palm oil, palm wine, soap, cloth, pots, firewood, the varied ingredients of charms and medicines, and European cloths and other imported items. They are dominated by women traders, the principal exception being the men who butcher and sell cattle from the north. During the day, before the market reaches its peak, women hawk their wares through town or sell them in front of the house and at street corners. Many women prepare and sell cooked food in the streets or scattered through the market. Over a century ago Bowen observed "No people are so much in the habit of eating in the streets, where women are always engaged in preparing all sorts of dishes for sale to passers by."*

MARKET SYSTEMS

West Africa, especially Yorubaland, but also the rest of the eastern part, is the most urbanized in Africa, a product no doubt of the higher level of commercial activity than in the rest of Africa. The Zaire River Basin also has a high level

---

*From *The Yoruba of Southwestern Nigeria* by William Bascom. Copyright © 1969 by Holt, Rinehart and Winston, Inc. Reprinted by permission of Holt, Rinehart and Winston.

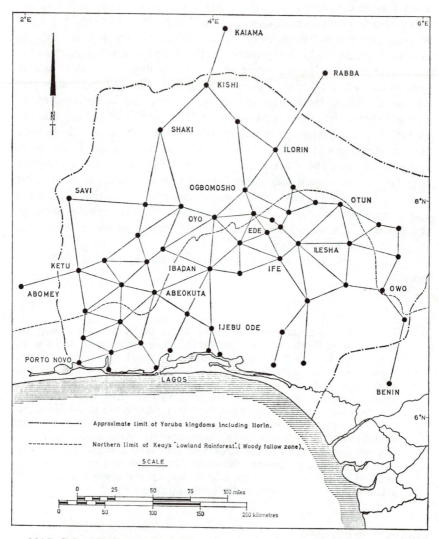

MAP 3.6 Major Yoruba Markets and Administrative Centers 1886
(from Morgan and Pugh, 1973)

of marketplace development. The rest of Africa contains only sporadic markets, if any. However, we should not confuse this with the existence of *market systems*. Market systems occur everywhere in Africa. A market system is one in which, to some appreciable degree, people depend on exchanging valuable things with others for things they want. Marketplaces are not necessary for this. Thus, for example, the most valuable rights sold by Africans everywhere are in their women—the marriage system. There are no market places where rights in women are sold, but all over Africa, arrangements are made for the exchange of rights in women, who ordinarily are absolutely essential for the operation of a homestead.

It is not possible to go into much detail about the importance of market and nonmarket trade in general, both within and between societies. Table 3.2 gives an indication of the amount of time people spend producing trade goods in one society (one-third of their time). We have already seen that Zaire is interlaced with trade routes. The foregoing account of periodic markets also is strong evidence of the generality of trade, in this case highly organized trade. Skinner (1962, 246), speaking of the Mossi of the western sudan, gives us another sample of nonmarket trade:

It is impossible to know the actual volume of caravan trade which passed through Mossi country, but we can get a fairly good idea of it by examining the customs reports on goods crossing the border between Mossi country and the northern territories of the Gold Coast in the few years just following European conquest. For 1901 and 1903 the official figures were

TABLE 3.2   Mossi Trade (1901–3)

YEAR	HORSES	CATTLE	SHEEP AND GOATS	LOADED DONKEYS	BALES OF COTTON CLOTH
1901	126	3,111	18,181	2,095	236
1903	196	6,624	30,892	4,294	369

Skinner continues:

Lucien Marc, who had the opportunity to check the volume of this trade for 1904 and 1905, guessed that about 16,000 cattle and 75,000 sheep and goats passed through the customs post in Mossi country. Furthermore, he believed that since . . . the Mossi also supply in part the markets of Togoland and the market at Bondoudou (Ivory Coast), one can estimate at least an annual export of 20,000 cattle and 100,000 sheep or goats. The import of kola nuts is at least 500 tons.

Another example of important nonmarket trade comes from early colonial Uganda (Driberg 1929). This involved the various ethnic groups of Acholi,

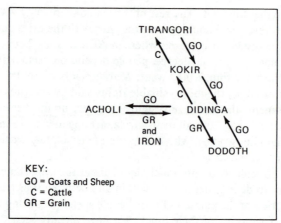

FIGURE 3.1 Long distance indigenous trade in
Northern Uganda
(from Driberg, 1929)

Didinga, Dodoth, Kokir, and Tirangori. The basis of this trade system was the
fact that each of these societies was trying to obtain a certain balance of grain,
livestock, and metal goods, but each was differentially successful in producing
one or the other. So, they traded directly and indirectly with each other to
balance their wants. Sometimes this required importing some things from
another society in order to trade these goods to a second society for more
desirable things. The Kokir bought goats from Tirangori (Figure 3.1) to the
north in return for cattle. The Kokir then traded the goats to the Didinga to
their south in return for cattle. The Didinga, in turn, shipped grain to *their*
south to get goats. Furthermore, the Didinga also traded goats to the Acholi
to their west to get grain and iron goods. A little reflection makes it plain that
what must be happening here is this: the Kokir are buying cattle from the
Didinga in order to resell to the Tirangori for a profit in goats, and they are
buying goats from the Tirangori to sell to the Didinga for a profit in cattle.
In other words, they are middlemen in the livestock trade. Similarly, the
Didinga are selling goats to the Acholi for grain in order to resell the grain
to the Dodoth for a profit. Looked at overall, this is an elaborate, interlocked,
"international" system in which goats, cattle, grain, and iron goods are being
redistributed to achieve a maximized balance of preferences, and the redistri-
bution is being accomplished by a profit system.

Suffice it to say that these examples are not unique although the volume
of marketing and level of production of market goods varies. In the cattle and
camel areas of East Africa, trade appears to have been less evident or of a
different order. Hence the lack of periodic markets associated with lower
populations. Furthermore, much wealth was tied up in large animals the

exchange of which was normally contractual, between parties whose claims on each other continued over long periods of time.

MONEY

This brings us to the matter of money. According with the fact that exchange activity within and between societies is universal is the fact of the nearly universal existence of money in one form or another. The kinds of currencies which occurred in Africa (and which still occur, since not all are obsolete) is very great. Einzig's book on "primitive" money (1966) lists the following things which served as media of exchange in one place or another in Africa: iron, salt, beads, cowry shells, calico cloth, cotton cloth, raffia palm cloth, slaves, gin, gold dust, brass rods, cattle, sheep, and goats. To this list may be added iron bars, brass bracelets, copper rods, and even oil (G. I. Jones 1977), in West Africa and Zaire, and muskets, powder, and shot in East Africa. It is important to understand what makes some good into a currency. First, it must be more highly valued than most other things. It does not matter in the least *why* the people value the good so long as they do. Thus for example, one might think that salt becomes a medium of exchange where it is rare because it is necessary to the human body. However, once the commodity takes on the role of money, with the flexibility it gives the holder for purchasing other goods, that fact changes people's views of salt money. It might now cease to be consumed and be used instead only for money. All African moneys are affected this way to some extent. For example, the iron knives which in some places in Zaire were used as money were produced in a conventionalized form; they could not actually be used as knives.

The second thing about a currency is that it must be cheap to keep. A highly valued commodity which cannot be easily transported and which costs a lot of resources just to preserve (such as grain) will not do. The reason crops seem almost never to serve as money is because they have value only in relatively large amounts, are perishable, and fluctuates widely in value between the preharvest and postharvest period. As the reader may readily imagine, if a repository of value maintains greater value relative to other goods, and if it is cheap to keep, it makes sense under many circumstances to convert other goods than money which are not immediately needed, into money where the value can be stored until needed. This explains why Africans are so desirous of obtaining domestic animals.

Although some kinds of money were widespread, not all were. Salt money, for example, seems to have had a very limited distribution, in the Horn of Africa, in particular. Similarly, cotton cloth functioned as money only in some places where it was produced or into which it was economical to trade

TABLE 3.3   Wolof Cloth Money—Equivalences of Cloth to Other Items (Ames 1962)

3 large kola nuts	1 xasap
6 handsful of unthreshed grain called a *sabarr*	1 xasap
8 *sabarr*	1 xopa
1 short handled hoe	2 xasap
1 rooster	2 xasap
1 large goat	1 xopa
1 cow	15 xopa
1 young female slave about 14 years old	20 xopa
Bridewealth payment (approximate)	32 xopa
1 horse	50 xopa

it, such as West Africa or southern Tanzania. The Arabs or coastal traders seem to have been responsible for introducing the loom and cotton into southern Tanzania, among the Fipa, in the eighteenth century, and their cloth served as money until the introduction of cloth from Europe, India, and America.

An especially interesting example of cloth money comes from the Wolof of the westernmost part of the western sudan (Ames 1955, 39). Table 3.3 indicates the terms for the money and the number of strips of cloth each stood for plus their value in British money in 1950. Table 3.4 shows some prices for various goods expressed in cloth money in 1950.

An example from East Africa of livestock used as money is found in the list on page 77, collected about 1910 in the Turu area of Tanzania by the German millitary commander of the District (Von Sick 1916).

TABLE 3.4   Wolof Cloth Money—Equivalences of Cloth (Ames 1962)

Wala wala or *sech* [*]	1 strip of cloth	3 pence
xasap	2 strips of cloth	6 pence
xasap and a *wala wala*	3 strips of cloth	9 pence
nyari (two) *xasap*	4 strips of cloth	1 shilling
nyari xasap and a *wala wala*	5 strips of cloth	1 shilling, 3 pence
nyeta xasap	6 strips of cloth	1 shilling, 6 pence
nyeta xasap and *wala wala*	7 strips of cloth	1 shilling, 9 pence
malan	8 strips of cloth	2 shillings
malan and a *wala wala*	9 strips of cloth	2 shillings, 3 pence
xopa	2 malan	4 shillings

[*] The *x* sound is like a k, as in king, and *e* like the e in bet.

10 goats = 1 steer
40 goats = 1 camel (hence four steers = one camel)
4 bags of grain (100–150 lbs) = 1 load of meat (two legs and a few other parts)
1 goat = 2 axes
1 goat = 1 spear
1 goat = a small irrigated plot; 2 goats = a large plot
1 goat = 1 pot of honey
1 steer = about Shs. 100 (in internal trade)
1 goat = about Shs. 10 (hence Shs. 100 = 10 goats = 1 steer)

Cowry shells obtained from the Indian Ocean were widely used in traditional Africa, both West and East. In West Africa, payments for rights in brides were quoted in some places in thousands of cowries, and cowries were the lowest denominator of currency in parts of East Africa. Bascom (1969, 27) says of Yoruba cowry money:

Although tradition speaks of a time when goods were bartered, for centuries, at least, money in the form of cowry shells was the basis of trade, and tradition also speaks of cowries being found in the lagoon. If the Yoruba did not have cowries before the Portuguese explored the coast, perhaps only in small numbers through trade from the Indian Ocean, one wonders what so quickly gave the Portuguese the idea that they were worth importing. In 1515 the King of Portugal issued a license to import cowry shells from India to Sao Tome; by 1522 they were being imported into Nigeria from the Malabar Coast, and during the seventeenth century from the East Indies. This resulted in their steady depreciation. In the middle of the nineteenth century the value of 2000 cowries was four shillings six pence, but it soon fell to less than two shillings when cheaper cowries were imported from Zanzibar. When cowries were replaced by coins, the value of 2000 cowries was stabilized at 6 pence for ritual purposes, or 80,000 to the pound sterling. Cowries were counted in strings of 40, in bunches of 200 (5 strings), in "heads" of 2000 (10 bunches), and in bags of 20,000 (10 heads) weighing 60 pounds.*

Raffia palm cloth appears to have had a very narrow range of distribution in Zaire. Gin was obviously a European introduction and was used as a medium of exchange in West Africa. Iron as money had a very wide distribution and was always a valuable commodity. African methods of smelting and working iron insured a relatively limited supply. Therefore, even working tools, such as hoe heads in East Africa, also served as money. Gold had a very limited distribution as money while brass rods seem to have been used only

*From *The Yoruba of Southwestern Nigeria* by William Bascom. Copyright © 1969 by Holt, Rinehart and Winston, Inc. Reprinted by permission of Holt, Rinehart and Winston.

in parts of Zaire and West Africa although brass wire was a currency in places in East Africa. Slaves, people in whom rights could be bought and sold, were a kind of human livestock in places where no large domestic animals could be raised, although they were not usually treated like livestock.

Of all the commodities serving as money in Africa, livestock, particularly cattle, was the most general and durable; it functions in this way even today among many Africans. It is often asserted that the African people do not eat their cattle. It would be truer to say that the animals are repositories of value and media of exchange, and to eat them would be equivalent to lighting your cigar with a ten dollar bill. In addition to their value as repositories of value, cattle have another sought after characteristic, shared only by certain other repositories of value—women, slaves, and other livestock—that they reproduce themselves. Cows are always the most valuable because they have calves. Thus, cattle are like money invested in stock, as our own ancestors knew since the words pecuniary, capital, and chattel all derive from livestock. They increase without further attention, although a more apt analogy is with bonds or savings accounts, the return from which is not erratic but relatively constant. It has been estimated that under average conditions of grazing, livestock disease, conception, and so on, fertile Zebu cows in Africa will double in a herd over nine and a half years (Dahl and Hjort 1976). Others have calculated a return on total herds of 20 percent a year. In addition, the rate of reproduction increases after famines when there is more grazing for individual animals.

That not only domestic animals have the ability to bring a return on an investment is indicated by credit institutions that flourish in many places, notably West Africa. Speaking again of the Yoruba, Bascom relates (1969, 27):

> Credit was available from money lenders at high rates of interest, through the institution of indenture or "pawning" and, since the introduction of cocoa, through the "pawning" of cocoa trees. It also was and is available through the *esusu,* an institution which has elements similar to installment buying, a credit union, and a savings club. The esusu is a fund to which a group of individuals make fixed contributions of money at fixed intervals; and the total amount contributed each period is assigned to each of the members in rotation. The number of contributors, the size of the contributions, and the length of the interval between contributions vary from one group to another; but if twenty members contribute one shilling each month at the end of twenty months, which completes the cycle, each member will have contributed one pound and received one pound in return. There is neither gain nor loss; but the advantage to the members is that they have one pound in a lump sum (or larger amounts of money if there are more members or larger contributions) with which to purchase goods, pay for services, or repay debts. Except for the one who receives the fund at the end of a cycle, all members receive an advance on their contributions without having to pay interest. Moreover, an

attempt is made to make the fund available to members at times when they have need for it, assigning it to a member who applies for it unless he has been tardy in making his payments or has already received the fund during the current cycle.*

SLAVERY

While the separation of material and social economy can be made with ease in most cases, trade of rights in persons brings us to a borderline example which demonstrates the ultimate inseparability of the two and the fact that society *is* economy.

Earlier in this chapter I referred in passing to Wolof cloth money and noted that Ames found that twenty xopa were equal to one young female slave. Africans had slavery, pawning, servitude—whatever one chooses to call it—except in the western sudan, perhaps, it was in many respects different from slavery as we know it in American history. In the Islamic areas of Africa, slaves usually formed a permanent endogenous (inmarrying) caste (MacGaffey 1978). Outside those areas, in the rest of Africa, they were more usually treated simply as people "without clans" who had been forceably or voluntarily removed from the context of their kin groups and attached to a lineage of masters to whom they were subordinate. Such persons could not own land and had no kinsmen to back them up. However, over several generations they could be absorbed by a master lineage, and slave women in many cases were even considered to be the best wives because they had no family to oppose the husband's wishes. Slaves could even own slaves.

Lest we conclude that African slavery was altogether benign, note that the Kongo people (MacGaffey 1970) classified them with witches in the sense that they had no clan while witches have betrayed their clans. Being on the margin of the social order (Vaughan 1977), so to speak, and having no one to claim blood money for them, they could be and were killed sometimes, for example, as sacrifices at the death of their masters. (Merriam [1974] questions whether slaves could be killed, at least among the Songye.)

Slavery seems not to occur among pastoral people, at least in East and southern Africa, whereas it may or may not occur in agricultural zones. This seems to be because slavery in the agricultural zones was equivalent to the raising of livestock in the pastoral zones. Slaves were repositories of value and could be used to effect exchanges, as in the Wolof case. They were also used extensively in some places in Central Africa for bridewealth, the payment for

---

*From *The Yoruba of Southwestern Nigeria* by William Bascom. Copyright © 1969 by Holt, Rinehart and Winston, Inc. Reprinted by permission of Holt, Rinehart and Winston.

a wife. Like cattle, slaves not only worked in the fields and so produced wealth, they also reproduced themselves. However slavery seems to have appeared only in the areas of greatest demand for labor, Central Africa and in spots in West Africa, or in the exceptional case in East Africa, as on the Kerebe Islands in Lake Victoria during the period when Arab demand for maize seems to have prompted the rise of slavery to meet the demand (Hartwig 1976). When cattle or camels can be raised, slavery has usually disappeared. Illustrating this point, Fielder (1973) tells us that the Ila of Zambia, who used to have slaves, turned very rapidly to agriculture with ox drawn plows (a capital intensive form of farming replacing the labor intensive form) when colonial authorities banned slavery. With the loss of slaves, the Ila found it economic to invest in agricultural capital where before, the use of slaves would have been less expensive. They found the opportunity cost worth the price since they had no alternative.

Lineages, that is to say, groups of kinsmen living together, are often not important in the pastoral zones because of the effects of high capital growth on the political economy, and for similar reasons slavery does not arise (a point that will be discussed more fully in later chapters). However, lineages are far more important in agricultural zones, and in a sense this is what makes slavery possible. Slavery removes a person who has no other resources from the protection of the lineage group.

Thus slavery in Africa is a kind of liminal process. Slaves can in some respects be thought of as simply human livestock, to be traded and even killed at the convenience of masters. But, on the other hand, they are also human beings, who can be married and even incorporated fully into a legitimate lineage. Therefore, what this demonstrates (as does the status of wife in many cases) is not that slavery was a marginal economic process, but that all exchanges including marriage or political support, are, like slavery, economic.

CONCLUSION

It will be useful, in closing this chapter, to stress an important fact about the relationship of production as a cultural trait to production and exchange as economic processes involving decisions about how much to produce and whether to exchange. There is no necessary correlation between the former and the latter. Two different people, both having knowledge of how to produce cattle, may nevertheless be unable to produce the same amounts. The one producing at a level giving a ratio of one cow per person will generate effects on the social system which the other cannot, as we shall see. Hence some cattle-raising people have matrilineality and states, and others do not. Similarly, among agricultural people, the low level of production of African cereals in Central Africa, or the high cost of production in that area, may be related to the widespread practice of matrilineality whereas in most other agricultural areas, matrilineality does not exist.

Finally, a word must be said about the currently popular subject of ecology. It has been noted by some students of the subject that there is a strong tendency for ethnic groups to be associated with particular habitats: the Kikuyu with the forests of the Aberdere Mountains on the east side of the Eastern Rift in Kenya; the Batswana with the low rainfall, high grasslands southeast of the Kalahari Desert; the Baganda with the fertile, well-watered belt of land on the north shore of Lake Victoria. The reason for this association, insofar as it exists (because it is not so clear-cut as sometimes claimed), is unclear. A popular idea is that it represents a kind of adjustment between an individual sociocultural system and the habitat, which serves the perpetuation of both, a balance which if disturbed brings about the degredation of each. I personally do not believe a case for this point of view can be supported. Habitat is always changing to one degree or another due to natural forces, like variations in rainfall and vegetation. Furthermore, the natural processes of the world are nowhere in static balance; societies or individuals do not seem to be so much in harmony with nature as in a standoff with it. Technology readjusts nature to fit human desires, the way prehistoric Africans cut over or eliminated the forests south of Lake Victoria or in the Zaire Basin. These activities have in some cases prepared conditions for the tsetse fly and have caused the elimination of domestic animals. Also, extensive grazing has often caused erosion and destruction of land by African pastoralists.

In other words, Africans, like ourselves, should be thought of as exploiters of the habitat for the general aim of increasing their wealth. In so doing they have, of course, caused problems for themselves, just as we have for ourselves.

MARRIAGE, DESCENT, AND ASSOCIATION

THE WAY HAVING BEEN PREPARED through the introduction of African material economics, we may now turn to the more general social sphere, what I earlier termed social exchange, the sphere of social economics. Marriage and descent are two subjects which have been central to the attention of social anthropologists for a very long time. In fact they were probably the main concern of British social anthropology. However, the mode of approach was mainly functionalist, as I explained in Chapter 1. From this perspective, marriage was seen almost as a ritual, rather than as an exchange act, and descent, arrangement of social groups in terms of relationship through the father or mother, was treated as a consequence of social rules, rather than as an economic process. Not much attention was paid to association probably because for functionalists, organization into descent groups and lineages and the reasons for this, were of prime theoretical interest.

To anticipate the discussion, we will find that marriage can be interpreted as an important exchange act designed to constitute a viable production unit by securing the main labor force. Descent of the unilineal kind, which is most prominent in Africa, is an important means of constituting large-scale labor cooperatives. Associations, on the other hand, will be seen as voluntary groupings of people to accomplish useful ends where descent groups are not possible or where they are no longer useful.

MARRIAGE

Unilineal Descent and Group Membership

Ethnologists speak of African societies as nearly universally displaying a pattern of *unilineal descent,* that is to say, *matrilineal descent,* as among the Yao of Mozambique, *patrilineal descent,* as among the Kipsigis of Kenya, or some combination of these, as among the Mbugwe of Tanzania whose system is sometimes referred to as *double descent.* In all these systems, descent is reckoned through *one* side of the parental generation, hence the *uni-* in unilineal descent. There is only one other way of reckoning descent in human societies, bilateral (or bilineal), as in the American system where descent is through both the mother and father, as shown by the fact that children inherit from both parents. However, it is an interesting contradictory fact that inheritance of surnames is patrilineal, the children taking their names from the father, not the mother.

While this may seem straightforward enough, the terms patrilineal and matrilineal in fact often represent two different, sometimes contradictory, things. When a society like the Ashanti of Ghana is called matrilineal, this usually means that membership in the most fundamental groups in the society is determined by the rule of matrilineal descent. A man is considered to be part of the group from which his mother, not his father, comes. He may not, in fact, live with his mother's group, but he is nevertheless part of it for such purposes as passing on to the next generation the property held by members of that group, wherever they may live. This is why these are often referred to as "descent groups." In the matrilineal case, the property of a man who has died passes to his sister's sons, and the property of a dead man in a patrilineal descent group passes to his sons.

As is apparent from a perusal of Map 4.1, the number of societies in Africa which may be described as having matrilineal descent groups is small, compared to those which are patrilineal. The largest grouping of matrilineal societies is in Central Africa, the so-called matrilineal belt. However, there is another important enclave in West Africa around and including the Ashanti.

8

Neurological Disorders

The complexity of anatomy and function of the nervous system results in confusion with the normal aging process and pathological processes. The most common health problems of the neurological system are presented in this chapter. Cerebrovascular accident, Parkinson's disease, and acute and chronic brain syndromes, including Alzheimer's disease, are discussed with special emphasis on rehabilitative measures.

CEREBROVASCULAR ACCIDENT

Cerebrovascular accident (CVA), or stroke, is the third leading cause of death in the aged, according to Podlone and Millikan (1981, p. 115). Cerebrovascular accident occurs when there is disruption of the brain's blood supply. The principal underlying cause of stroke is atherosclerotic changes in the vasculature of the brain. Dehydration, diabetes, anemia, and hypertension can be predisposing causes of stroke. Signs and symptoms of stroke include aphasia, visual disturbances, hemiplegia, and sensory changes. Symptoms may last only a few minutes or hours; these episodes are known as transient ischemic attacks (TIAs). They often occur before a major stroke.

The severity of the stroke depends upon the area of the brain and the amount of brain tissue involved. Damage to the

3. A method of assessing vertebral compression associated with osporosis is to measure from _____ _____ and to compare the measurement to the person's height.

4. _____ generally involves joint deformity and intense pain.

5. The first consideration when a person sustains a fractured hip is _____ .